MORTEN SKOVDAL

PARADOXES OF PrEP FOR HIV PREVENTION

POLICY PRESS SHORTS POLICY & PRACTICE

First published in Great Britain in 2025 by

Policy Press, an imprint of
Bristol University Press
University of Bristol
1–9 Old Park Hill
Bristol
BS2 8BB
UK
t: +44 (0)117 374 6645
e: bup-info@bristol.ac.uk

Details of international sales and distribution partners are available at
policy.bristoluniversitypress.co.uk

© Morten Skovdal 2025

The digital PDF and EPUB versions of this title are available open access and distributed under the terms of the Creative Commons Attribution 4.0 International licence (https://creativecommons.org/licenses/by/4.0/) which permits adaptation, alteration, reproduction, and distribution without further permission provided the original work is attributed.

British Library Cataloguing in Publication Data
A catalogue record for this book is available from the British Library

ISBN 978-1-4473-7536-4 paperback
ISBN 978-1-4473-7250-9 ePub
ISBN 978-1-4473-7251-6 OA PDF

The right of Morten Skovdal to be identified as author of this work has been asserted by him in accordance with the Copyright, Designs and Patents Act 1988.

All rights reserved: no part of this publication may be reproduced, stored in a retrieval system, or transmitted in any form or by any means, electronic, mechanical, photocopying, recording, or otherwise without the prior permission of Bristol University Press.

Every reasonable effort has been made to obtain permission to reproduce copyrighted material. If, however, anyone knows of an oversight, please contact the publisher.

The statements and opinions contained within this publication are solely those of the author and not of the University of Bristol or Bristol University Press. The University of Bristol and Bristol University Press disclaim responsibility for any injury to persons or property resulting from any material published in this publication.

Bristol University Press and Policy Press work to counter discrimination on grounds of gender, race, disability, age, and sexuality.

Cover design: Bristol University Press
Front cover image: Alamy Stock Photo/Bowonpat Sakaew
Bristol University Press and Policy Press use environmentally responsible print partners.
Printed and bound in Great Britain by CPI Group (UK) Ltd, Croydon, CR0 4YY

Contents

List of figures, tables, and boxes		iv
Preface		v
one	PrEP for HIV prevention	1
two	The case studies	24
three	Free, yet costly	48
four	Eligible, yet ineligible	60
five	Responsible, yet irresponsible	78
six	Healthy, yet a patient	97
seven	Safe, yet unsafe	114
eight	Liberating, yet constraining	126
nine	PrEP paradoxes: problematic, yet productive	142
Notes		156
References		157
Index		172

List of figures, tables, and boxes

Figures
1.1	The social representations paradox model	21
2.1	'Picturing PrEP' exhibition	39
3.1	More than a glass of water	50
4.1	Fear of judgement from parents	62
4.2	A church poster	64
5.1	Condom	81
5.2	Rejected by people on PrEP	84
5.3	Talking to friends	91
6.1	Pills, more pills	100
6.2	The hospital	101
6.3	The pharmacy	104
6.4	Pills	110
7.1	PrEP and party and play	120
8.1	'How long should I take PrEP for?'	137

Tables
2.1	PrEP services in Zimbabwe and Denmark	33
2.2	Study participant characteristics	37
2.3	Thematic network table of findings	42

Boxes
1.1	Definition of 'everyday PrEP negotiations'	20

Preface

The story of this book is rather simple. It is a story about people being pensive about oral pre-exposure prophylaxis (PrEP) for HIV prevention. It is a story about how contrary ideas and 'ways of thinking' about PrEP complicate PrEP uptake and utilisation. I will tell it as a classic social psychological story, focusing on the dynamic interactions that exist between social context and individual thoughts, feelings, and actions related to PrEP. The book draws on research from two qualitative studies that sought to generate a user perspective on PrEP, and thus offers a comparative perspective between different target groups (queer men vs young straight women) and contexts (Global North vs Global South). The study with queer men was conducted in Denmark and funded by AIDS-Fondet (the Danish AIDS Foundation). The study with young heterosexual women in Zimbabwe was jointly funded by the US National Institutes of Mental Health (R01MH114562–01) and the Bill and Melinda Gates Foundation (INV-009999). The Bill and Melinda Gates Foundation kindly agreed to waive the open access fees of this book, for which I am very grateful. It is important to note that the content in this book does not necessarily represent the official views of the funders.

The research and findings presented in the book did not magically emerge from raw data. They reflect many years of collaborative work and thinking, for which I am deeply indebted. First, I would like to acknowledge and express my deep gratitude and indebtedness to Professor Catherine

ONE

PrEP for HIV prevention

This is a book about PrEP, which refers to a cluster of pharmaceutical medications that can prevent the human immunodeficiency virus (HIV) from taking hold in people who have been exposed to the virus. A PrEP prescription typically involves regular visits to a health facility, both to determine PrEP candidacy and to ascertain health by screening and monitoring for sexually transmitted infections and kidney function. Although different modes of PrEP administration are beginning to emerge, oral PrEP, the swallowing of a PrEP pill (typically Truvada) either daily or on demand – meaning before and after sex – remains the most common method. Oral PrEP, the focus of this book, is over 99 per cent effective at preventing HIV when correctly adhered to.

This brief opening alludes to one of the six paradoxes covered in this book, namely that a PrEP user is *both* healthy *and* a patient. I have constructed this paradox and others in the book to produce seemingly contradictory statements. This is also captured by the chapter titles. I do this both to challenge assumptions and to make visible the complex realities of PrEP use. People either interested in or already using PrEP will inevitably encounter conflictual ideas about it. A PrEP user may feel healthy and know that their access to PrEP is conditional on good health. Health screenings and monitoring are in place to confirm their health and eligibility. All the same, the PrEP treatment regimen requires daily pill-taking and occasional visits to health facilities, which the same individual may associate strongly with illness and being a patient. This can lead to a sense of ambiguity whereby the individual fluctuates between the sensation of feeling healthy or like a patient. In the context of PrEP, conflicting and contradictory ideas are plentiful and often encountered in everyday life. They do not go unnoticed and contribute to contentions, uncertainties, dilemmas, and ambiguities that need to be carefully and pensively responded to through processes that I term 'everyday PrEP negotiations'. My analysis indicates that the nature and need for such everyday PrEP negotiations play an instrumental role in explaining people's varying abilities to engage with PrEP and why PrEP works for some people and not for others. I will therefore also draw attention to the factors that mediate and determine the need for everyday PrEP negotiations. This includes highlighting the social construction of conflicting and contradictory ideas, and how they are both an outcome of shared beliefs and understandings, and amenable to change and reconstruction through participation in social groups and networks. This allows me to point to areas of intervention.

Though not a topic we set out to research, different 'ways of thinking' about PrEP are omnipresent in the studies that my colleagues and I have been working on for the past seven years. Here we have had the privilege of working with adolescent girls and young women in Zimbabwe and queer men in Denmark to understand their perspectives on and experiences of PrEP. Although other researchers have alluded to PrEP paradoxes in article formats (for example, Knight et al., 2016), I decided to present an analysis of the role of paradoxes in PrEP use in book form. I did this both to capture and collate the sheer number of paradoxes identifiable in our data material, and to understand similarities and differences in how paradoxes manifest and come to determine PrEP use in two very different countries and with two distinct groups whose allegiances to social identities, group norms, and cultural traditions differ significantly. A key tenet of the book is therefore that what our participants say about PrEP, and the different ideas and ways of thinking they articulate, are inherently social in nature and can only be fully understood by considering their social and cultural context.

Through this social lens, I hope that this book can offer prevention researchers, planners, and evaluators new insights and an analytical tool to recognise and respond to the social context of PrEP use. It is also my hope that PrEP users who read this book will find comfort in the recognition of the complexities and social nature of their everyday PrEP negotiations. I also hope they will feel inspired to participate in community-oriented interventions that counter and reformulate unhelpful and conflictual ideas, making it easier to take up PrEP and making it work for more people.

For the remainder of this introductory chapter, I will expand both on my aims in writing this book and on the book's significance for the field of HIV prevention, and for biomedical prevention more broadly. This will involve providing more context to the global HIV response and the need to intensify prevention efforts. Then I will expand on the role of PrEP in these efforts. There then follows a more detailed discussion of what can be done to maximise the impact of PrEP, making PrEP work for more people. This includes highlighting some controversies that surround PrEP and that obstruct uptake and utilisation. Before briefly introducing each of the chapters, I present the conceptual framework guiding my writing and analysis.

A case of biomedical prevention

PrEP is just one of a rapidly expanding list of preventive medicines that can help people avoid certain illnesses or conditions. Preventive medicine is something we are all familiar with and benefit greatly from. You have most likely received several vaccinations in your lifetime, perhaps most recently to prevent, or at least boost immunity to, COVID-19. If you are a woman, you may well have experience of using hormonal contraceptives to prevent unwanted pregnancy. Perhaps you have travelled to regions where malaria is prevalent and been prescribed antimalarial drugs to prevent infection. If your cholesterol levels are high, you may be prescribed medications such as statins to reduce the risk of cardiovascular diseases. More recently, weight loss medications have received much attention for their transformative potential and for being in high demand.

I relate PrEP to the growing list of preventive medicines for two reasons. The first is to position this book within the broader field of biomedical prevention, where there are many common challenges with regards to adherence, access, affordability, risk perception and awareness, side effects or concerns about safety, and issues of implementation and distribution. Findings from this book, as well as the conceptual tools and language arising in this work, are hopefully applicable to other preventive medicine contexts. This brings me to the second reason: to engage you, the reader, and to encourage you to help me relate the applicability of PrEP paradoxes to other preventive medicines. As you read, I invite you to draw parallels between the paradoxes and findings presented in this book (about PrEP) and your own experiences with preventive medicine or preventive technologies more broadly (for example, hearing aid use in people with hearing loss to reduce risk of dementia). What negotiations took place before you made the decision to engage with the prevention method? What were your considerations? What did the method require of you? What work was involved in using it?

As you go through the book, it may become clear how your own negotiations of risks, benefits, and social acceptability involves considering opposing and conflictual ideas, cultural values, social norms, and practices. Hopefully, this approach will help cement the relevance of this book beyond HIV and

PrEP. However, HIV and PrEP make a particularly instructive case study. As HIV is intrinsically linked to issues of sexuality, stigma, and structural disparities such as poverty, race, or gender, this book arguably constitutes what Flyvbjerg (2006) calls an 'extreme case'. It thus activates actors and mechanisms that make the paradoxes more pronounced. While the paradoxes will manifest differently between health and disease contexts, and other paradoxes may apply, it is my hope that this book will begin to demarcate paradoxes and their constitutive relationship with biomedical prevention negotiations as a specific problem space for research and practice in preventive medicine.

HIV, global targets, and the need to intensify prevention efforts

Despite extraordinary gains in making effective HIV treatment available, HIV remains a leading cause of death worldwide. For women of reproductive age, HIV is *the* leading cause of death (UNAIDS, 2019). In 2021, an estimated 650,000 persons succumbed needlessly to acquired immune deficiency syndrome (AIDS) (UNAIDS, 2022b). That is one person every minute. In the same year, 1.5 million people acquired HIV, with new HIV infections rising in many communities and countries (UNAIDS, 2022b). Although these numbers represent a significant reduction from the mortality and infection rates at the height of the global HIV epidemic in the late 1990s, current infection rates are still substantially off global targets, which aimed for fewer than 500,000 new cases by 2020 (UNAIDS, 2014). The current state of the global HIV epidemic is disappointing, not least given the optimism and ambitious targets that have characterised much of the global HIV response over the past decade. Personally, I vividly remember the enthusiasm and hopefulness that characterised the 19th International AIDS Conference in 2012, held in Washington, DC under the theme 'Turning the Tide Together'.[1] The main message of the conference was that we now have the solutions and tools to end the HIV epidemic, and the global community must work together to end the spread of HIV. The conference took place at a time of substantial scientific breakthroughs, with advances being made in the range and efficacy of HIV prevention technologies. In addition to PrEP, this included treatment as prevention, which refers to the use of antiretroviral treatment to lower the risk of HIV transmission. People living with HIV who consistently adhere to their antiretroviral treatment can reach undetectable levels of viral load, which prevents them from transmitting HIV to their sexual partners (Cohen et al., 2011). Voluntary medical male circumcision also proved efficacious, lowering men's risk of HIV infection by up to 60 per cent (Auvert et al., 2005).

On the back of these biomedical discoveries, and the political commitments and global solidarity present at the time, new targets saw the light of day. The Fast-Track approach to end the AIDS epidemic as a public health threat was introduced in 2014. It included the 90–90–90 treatment targets (by 2020, 90 per cent of people living with HIV should know their HIV status; by 2020, 90 per cent of people who know their HIV status should be on treatment; by 2020, 90 per cent of people on treatment should achieve viral suppression), which have been widely adopted and largely successful in accelerating access to testing and treatment services worldwide. It also included primary HIV prevention targets, such as 90 per cent of boys and men (aged 10–29) in countries with generalised HIV epidemics getting circumcised; 90 per cent of people at elevated risk of HIV having access to a combination of prevention programmes; and 90 per cent of those people at particularly elevated risk reporting condom use at last sex act (Stover et al., 2016). These different Fast-Track targets have since been increased to 95% (UNAIDS, 2022a).

According to recent calculations of data available up until 2020, eight countries with very different epidemics (Eswatini, Rwanda, Qatar, Botswana, Slovenia, Uganda, Malawi, and Switzerland) have either achieved or gone beyond the 90–90–90 treatment targets (Frescura et al., 2022). Many more countries are expected to follow in the years to come. Wonderful as this is, the continuing high, and often rising, rates of HIV infection indicate challenges to the realisation of some of the assumptions guiding the HIV prevention potential of the Fast-Track targets. For starters, at a population level, treatment as prevention has proved less effective (in real-life settings) than hoped for, with either no (Iwuji et al., 2018) or a less than 30% reduction in incidence (Hayes et al., 2019; Makhema et al., 2019). In other words, the successes in scaling up testing and treatment services are not translating into significant reductions in HIV transmission. Furthermore, it has been suggested that financial investments to achieve the prevention targets have been lower than required. All this combined spurs calls to further maximise the impact of primary prevention methods, such as condoms, male circumcision, and PrEP (Ward et al., 2019). This book seeks to support this agenda, albeit from a social science perspective.

The promises and perils of PrEP

Oral PrEP is being hailed as one of the best prevention methods at our disposal to end HIV transmission. HIV activists and researchers often refer to oral PrEP as 'revolutionary' and a 'game-changer' for HIV prevention; a 'miracle drug' that can end the deadliest epidemic of modern times. And for very good reason. A recent systematic review and meta-analysis of the 15 trials conducted to date establishes the effectiveness of PrEP (Murchu et al., 2022). It finds that PrEP is highly effective, particularly among men who have sex with men and serodiscordant couples (where one partner lives with HIV and the other does not). In fact, when PrEP is widely used and adhered to – which is the case among certain pockets of the queer community, predominantly in the White, urban Global North – it can lead to significant population-level reductions in new HIV infections. Examples of PrEP-led successes towards epidemic control have been observed in the

UK (Girometti et al., 2021; Sullivan et al., 2023), Australia (Grulich et al., 2021), and the US (Smith et al., 2020). While this is encouraging, many population groups at risk of HIV do not benefit from the promises of PrEP. The review by Murchu et al. also finds that none of the five trials conducted with heterosexual women in sub-Saharan Africa – a group at high risk of HIV – demonstrate a reduction in HIV acquisition because of PrEP. This is explained by low levels of uptake and adherence (Van Damme et al., 2012; Marrazzo et al., 2015), and suggests that women in parts of sub-Saharan Africa face particular gendered challenges in their engagement with PrEP, something this book explores in detail. Other groups face difficulties too. Countless PrEP implementation studies are reporting on barriers to PrEP access and adherence among different groups vulnerable to HIV – including trans persons, sex workers, prisoners, people who inject drugs, and migrants – in a variety of countries (Murchu et al., 2022). Furthermore, and as alluded to earlier, gay, bisexual, and other men who have sex with men are not a homogenous group. In the US, Black and Latinx men who have sex with men, for instance, have lower levels of PrEP uptake, and studies are looking to identify and respond to the many inequities that prevent many gay men of colour from engaging with PrEP effectively (Rolle et al., 2017; Taggart et al., 2020).

Maximising the impact of PrEP

It is evident that PrEP works very well for some people, but not for most people vulnerable to HIV. As long as this is the case, the 'game-changing' potential of PrEP to bend the curve of the global HIV epidemic remains unfulfilled. This raises the question: How do we maximise the impact of PrEP? There is clearly not a single right answer to this question. The question was discussed in relation to HIV prevention technologies at a small meeting of experts hosted by the Bill and Melinda Gates Foundation at Cold Spring Harbor

Laboratory's science think tank in 2017. I participated in the meeting, and unsurprisingly we concluded that many different elements need to come together. We identified community engagement and social marketing, participation and ownership, integrated health services and choice, and solid evidence and data as some of the core elements (Ward et al., 2019). That said, three approaches to maximise the impact of PrEP appear to predominate over HIV prevention research and innovation, cementing the dominance of biomedical, implementation, and health services research.

The first approach seeks to biomedically innovate our way out of challenges. This work rides on the wave of scientific breakthroughs within biomedical science to develop and deploy an ever-expanding range of efficacious biomedical technologies. In addition to oral PrEP, other PrEP products that have recently been approved for use include a vaginal silicone ring, which, when inserted into the vagina, slowly releases an antiretroviral drug and offers protection against HIV over a 30-day period. Injectable PrEP has also been approved and is slowly being rolled out. Here individuals vulnerable to HIV can choose to receive a PrEP injection every two months. Other HIV prevention technologies in the pipeline[2] include dissolvable or removable implants that slowly dissolve PrEP medication into the body, longer-acting oral PrEP pills, and dual prevention pills (combining PrEP with oral contraceptives). Each new PrEP product responds to implementation challenges of oral PrEP. Another guiding assumption behind the expanding number of PrEP products is that by providing people with different tools and more choices, they are much more likely to find a combination of methods that works for them, and that this is critical to fill the prevention gap. It is inevitable that some of these new PrEP products will productively respond to some of the challenges to oral PrEP outlined in this book, and I emphasise: this book celebrates these remarkable advances. However, they bear witness to a biomedical turn in HIV prevention – one that may reduce HIV prevention to pill-taking, implants, and injectables delivered through standard, clinic-based models of care. While it is easy to be seduced by such technological fixes, they assume that health services have the capacity (knowledge, time, and resources) to be able to counsel and deliver a range of different prevention modalities to different population groups, *and* that people are autonomous and rational actors with unfettered access to these services. According to Bernays et al. (2021), a real danger of this strong biomedical approach to PrEP and HIV prevention more broadly is that it undermines and blurs the visibility of social influences.

Challenges in access to oral PrEP have cemented the significance of a second approach – one that is more health service- and implementation-focused – namely, to understand how community-centred and simplified health services can shape behaviours and engagement with PrEP. This work recognises the limits of standard, clinic-based models of HIV prevention care in reaching the most vulnerable and difficult to reach. It includes work around community-based interventions to reach underserved groups and foster demand for and sustained engagement with PrEP. It also includes efforts to differentiate health services so that they can adapt to the needs and preferences of different population segments, or profiles of people who could benefit from PrEP. The most recent PrEP implementation guidelines from the World Health Organization demonstrate this approach (WHO, 2022). The guidelines adapt the differentiated service delivery framework and encourage service providers to be more flexible when it comes to *when* a PrEP service is delivered, *where* it is delivered, *what* is being delivered, and *who* delivers it. The power of more differentiated and simplified service delivery became clear during the COVID-19 pandemic, when service providers who adapted their PrEP service delivery in response to pandemic restrictions began to observe a surge in the demand for PrEP. For instance, some adopted telemedicine solutions, and this change in *where* PrEP services are delivered was noted to increase the number of people on PrEP in a variety of contexts (Dourado et al., 2020; Rogers et al., 2020; Hill et al., 2021; Kerzner et al., 2022). When COVID-19 restrictions were in place in Zimbabwe, PrEP services for female sex workers shifted from clinical settings towards community, home-based, and peer-led PrEP services, and these shifts in *where* and *who* delivers PrEP meant that PrEP use 'went through the roof' (Matambanadzo et al., 2021).

A third approach to maximise the impact of PrEP draws on systems thinking and complexity theory to integrate PrEP within a layer of other interventions. This work is referred to as 'combination HIV prevention' and is supported by solid research that documents the added value of combining interventions (Cluver et al., 2016; Toska et al., 2017). It assumes that there is no single magic bullet to end the HIV epidemic, but that a combination of biomedical, behavioural, and structural interventions, carefully packaged to match the profile of a target population, will take us an important step further (Kurth et al., 2011). The Determined, Resilient, Empowered, AIDS-free, Mentored, and Safe (DREAMS) partnership is arguably the largest and most well-known example of a combination HIV prevention initiative involving PrEP. DREAMS seeks to reduce new HIV diagnoses among adolescent girls and young women in ten sub-Saharan African countries. The programme contains a core package of 13 interventions, of which PrEP is one. The underlying assumption behind DREAMS is what when layers of biomedical, behavioural, or structural interventions are introduced, targeting different groups (the young women themselves, family members, their male partners, and the broader community), synergies will emerge, contributing to greater and longer-lasting impacts (Saul et al., 2018). Evaluations of DREAMS are beginning to emerge. While the evidence is mixed, greater declines in new HIV diagnoses are observed in settings where more DREAMS interventions are implemented (Saul et al., 2022). Some DREAMS sites have experienced difficulties and delays in the implementation of community-based norms interventions (Gourlay et al., 2019), which may explain variances in reductions. The DREAMS partnership laudably responds to some of the social, political, economic, and environmental factors that determine adolescent girls' and young women's vulnerability to HIV and their various different abilities to confront HIV. However, a criticism of how combination HIV prevention is often implemented in practice, which I have raised elsewhere, is that the justifications for bringing together a set layer of interventions are often weak and unclear. It is notoriously difficult to ascertain exactly what layers of interventions to combine in order to increase their synergistic effects (Skovdal, 2019). While responding with evidence-informed interventions at different levels is likely to be beneficial, doing so without an interrogation of *how* the interventions interact in (and with) a particular context and make PrEP work, or not, for people may undermine otherwise comprehensive prevention combination programmes. Auerbach and Hoppe (2015: p 1) argue that the quest for ways to 'get drugs into bodies', which is a principle present in the three approaches mentioned earlier, often renders social context and its ability to make PrEP work for people invisible. This calls for a fourth approach.

Towards making PrEP work for people in their everyday lives

While new PrEP products and more person-centred service delivery options are central to making the work involved with PrEP more manageable and doable, their success will depend on recognising and working with the reality of people's everyday lives. A fourth approach would thus seek to understand and respond to what it takes to get PrEP to *work for* people in their everyday lives (Kippax, 2012; Auerbach and Hoppe, 2015; Skovdal, 2019). For me, and to continue the work metaphor, this first and foremost entails an understanding of the *work involved* in using PrEP and how PrEP *works on* individuals and communities. If individuals and communities have found ways to make the work manageable, and PrEP affects their lives positively and meaningfully, then PrEP fits into their everyday lives and works for them. On the contrary, if the work involved is draining, risky, or obstructs their everyday lives, and affects individuals or a community negatively, PrEP is unlikely to work for them.

The relevance of considering the 'work involved' is captured by the expanding *patient* work literature that has emerged within health sociology, with roots in Corbin and Strauss's (1985) seminal piece on chronic illness management. The concept of patient work has been instrumental in making visible the efforts and activities of patients that are otherwise taken for granted yet are key to the success of their treatment (Yin et al., 2020). Corbin and Strauss (1985) themselves note illness-related work (for example, diagnosis, medicine-taking, symptom management), everyday life work (for example, raising children, keeping a marriage and a household going), and biographical work (for example, making sense of the illness, identity formation, dealing with significant life events) as overarching lines of work that affect illness management. Many other types of work have since been identified, such as care navigation work (Defty et al., 2023), time management work (Jowsey et al., 2012), and work with digital health technologies (Leese et al., 2022).

However, the patient work literature is – for good reasons – almost exclusively focused on people living with chronic conditions. As noted by Haaland et al. (2023), the work of people preventing illness is rarely studied. This book speaks directly to this gap. It builds on work that Primdahl and I have published elsewhere, where we report on six categories of work that queer men in Denmark activate to access and utilise PrEP. These include: *work out* the system of PrEP access; identify *what works* to access PrEP; w*orking* PrEP services to their advantage; *work with* the PrEP service delivery system; *work through* what it means to be on PrEP; and *work for* PrEP visibility (Primdahl and Skovdal, 2023). In a Tanzanian context, Haaland et al. (2023) note three types of PrEP patient work: the practical efforts of getting enrolled onto a PrEP programme (readying work), adhering to PrEP (user work), and managing the disclosure of their PrEP use in a social context (social navigation work). With the exception of a few examples from the disease management literature (Bagge-Petersen et al., 2020; Gammeltoft et al., 2022; Bagge-Petersen, 2023), little has been done to understand what work goes into dealing with the contentions, uncertainties, dilemmas, and ambiguities arising from opposing and conflicting interests and ideas. It is my hope that this book can help further advance the visibility of such work, albeit in the context of prevention medicine.

PrEP also *works on* people in different ways. Social scientists are beginning to document the different ways PrEP leaches into people's social lives, mediating relationship dynamics and how sex is experienced and practised (Dean, 2015; Young et al., 2016; Brisson and Nguyen, 2017; García-Iglesias, 2022; Primdahl and Skovdal, 2023). Such work adopts a post-humanist perspective and recognises the agency of the PrEP pill (and social practices associated with pill-taking) in dynamically shaping how PrEP users live their lives. This book contributes to this expanding social science literature, making way for stories that illuminate how PrEP uptake and utilisation are mediated by either considerations or experiences of how PrEP affects people's social and sexual lives, and indeed identities.

By way of introduction to some of the social dimensions that give rise to different representations and ways of thinking and talking about PrEP, I now turn to a discussion of some of the controversies that circulate in society about PrEP. This both provides background to some of the findings presented in the forthcoming chapters, and offers a segue to the conceptual framework that guides my analysis and writing.

PrEP and moral responsibilities for (un)healthy behaviours

PrEP has – perhaps more than any other preventive medicine – been immersed in controversy and public criticism. This controversy is rooted in moral values and judgements about who should take responsibility for risk. The controversies tend to be about whether the moral responsibility for preventing HIV rests with the individual or society. What further complicates this issue is the controversy associated with spending public resources on a preventive drug, which necessitates a consideration or intention of risk. If this risk-taking is by a marginalised and stigmatised group, such as gay men, people who inject drugs, or sex workers, they are likely to be further vilified for their so-called risky practices. To exemplify this, let me briefly highlight some of the controversies arising from the slow PrEP roll-out in England. They are well documented in the British press and academic literature and lucidly discussed in the BBC documentary 'The People vs The NHS: Who Gets the Drugs?'[3].

PrEP was only made freely available through the UK's National Health Service (NHS) in 2020, eight years after the drug was initially approved for HIV prevention by the US Food and Drug Administration. Until then, access to PrEP was limited to individuals participating in the national PrEP Impact Trial, or with the means to buy the branded drug Truvada privately (around £400/month) or generic equivalents online from overseas sellers (around £45/month). The 'battle' to get PrEP rolled out on the NHS was arduous, and involved the National AIDS Trust, a UK-based charity, taking NHS England to court and winning, claiming that it is within the power of NHS England to fund PrEP. The initial NHS England decision not to fund PrEP was due to the high cost of PrEP and the NHS's claim that HIV prevention is the job of local councils (Hawkes, 2016). This battle played out in the British press, igniting views about the supposed immorality of 'promiscuous', 'unsafe', and homosexual sex. In an analysis of how the British press discussed and represented PrEP, Mowlabocus (2020) notes the common use of terms such as 'Truvada whores', the 'promiscuity pill', and the 'lifestyle drug', particularly in the right-wing press. These metaphors constitute useful codes for communicating and emphasising individual responsibility and choice. They qualify several claims and fears. According to Mowlabocus, this includes the claim that PrEP, if offered by the NHS, will incentivise and subsidise the reckless sexual behaviours of gay men. A related claim was that support of such a 'lifestyle drug' would result in resources being taken away from the treatment of children and old people. NHS England confirmed this narrative by releasing statements about how PrEP will prohibit certain treatments (and unnecessarily stressed that PrEP is used by men who have sex with men) (NHS England, 2016). Another claim raised in the press was that PrEP may lead to more promiscuity and more condomless anal sex, which in turn may give rise to increases in sexually transmitted infections, affecting the broader public negatively. The view that gay men should take more personal responsibility, either by using condoms – the cheaper alternative – or by paying for PrEP themselves, was common (Mowlabocus, 2020).

Before I continue, I would like to debunk some of the views and fears described earlier. Research demonstrates that the HIV response cannot rely on condoms or any other single prevention method. While condoms are critical to the HIV response, they are often used inconsistently (Smith et al., 2015). Combining HIV prevention methods yields the greatest impact (Lasry et al., 2014; Pickles et al., 2023). PrEP has also proved highly cost-effective by reducing healthcare-related expenditures associated with HIV treatment (Cambiano et al., 2018; Durand-Zaleski et al., 2018). A recent review on the effectiveness and safety of PrEP found no evidence of increases in sexually transmitted infections (Murchu et al., 2022). In fact, a growing number of real-world, population-level studies are observing declines in sexually transmitted infections, possibly due to the increases in testing for sexually transmitted infections among queer men on PrEP (Morgan et al., 2020; Traeger et al., 2022). Furthermore, a review by Kojima et al. (2016), which claimed that PrEP contributes to high rates of sexually transmitted infections among men who have sex with men, was quickly discredited on scientific grounds (Harawa et al., 2017). When associations between PrEP use and increases in the overall incidence of sexually transmitted infections have been found, this is often due to increases preceding PrEP initiation. This has been found in Denmark and is indicative of queer men seeking out PrEP during periods where there is a growing chance of them contracting a sexually transmitted infection (von Schreeb et al., 2024). Such findings should alleviate concerns that PrEP automatically leads to increases in sexually transmitted infections.

Despite such evidence, the viewpoints and fears discussed earlier continue to circulate in the public sphere – not just in England, but everywhere. They are value-laden and almost always echoing many past and ongoing struggles in the HIV response, reflecting views around moral and sexual conduct. They may, however, take different forms. In countries with a tax-funded national health service, debates about individual responsibility may be more forthright. In countries with a strong patriarchal culture, and where gender orders prohibit the sexual autonomy of adolescent girls and young women, debates and fears about how PrEP may lead to more sexual independence among women may dominate. As I will demonstrate in this book, the collective and common symbols, meanings, ideas, values, norms, and practices about PrEP that circulate in different social milieus matter hugely and form the foundation for many of the paradoxes that characterise PrEP. They complicate access and engagement with PrEP in ways we do not yet fully understand.

I now turn to the conceptual framework that will help me disentangle how collective and common ways of thinking and talking about PrEP heighten the need for everyday PrEP negotiations and affect PrEP use.

My conceptual lens

First, I must state that I am a social psychologist with a keen interest in community levels of analysis. I therefore approach the individual as someone who stands in a mutually constitutive relationship with the social world they inhabit. I will therefore not focus on bigger structural problems or rely on individual capacities, such as perceptions of HIV vulnerability or attitudes, to explain variances in PrEP uptake and utilisation. Social scientists from other disciplines are already doing a fantastic job in highlighting individual and structural determinants of PrEP use. I will of course touch on these issues, as they form part of the bigger story, but only to show how they interact and come together at a community level to shape the shared ideas, values, norms, and practices that determine how people encounter, respond to, and negotiate PrEP use in their everyday life.

To help me do this I turn to social representations theory (SRT). SRT was developed by Moscovici (1973) to understand everyday ways of thinking, and the stock of ideas that enable people to navigate the social world and to communicate with people about it. According to Joffe (2002), SRT is particularly useful for research with an interest in the social, emotive and symbolic facets of health. Moscovici has characterised social representations like this:

> [as] systems of values, ideas and practices with a twofold function: first to establish an order which will enable individuals to orientate themselves in their material and social world and to master it; and secondly to enable communication to take place among the members of a community by providing them with a code for social exchange and a code for naming and classifying unambiguously the various aspects of their world and their individual and group history. (Moscovici, 1973: p xiii)

Put differently, social representations refer to the ideas and ways of thinking that are attached to PrEP, such as it being expensive or linked to promiscuity. Other examples were mentioned in the previous section. These ideas and ways of thinking determine how people communicate about PrEP, make sense of it, and engage with it. A key tenet of SRT is that these ideas and ways of thinking are always constructed and given meaning through interactions and exchanges of ideas between the self and others (Marková, 2003). As such, what the ideas and ways of thinking are, their symbolic meanings, and how they dialogically enter people's lives and come to affect thoughts and actions around PrEP use, will differ between social milieus.

However, this also means that people taking, or interested in, PrEP are bound to encounter diverging views and opposing perspectives depending on the social context they find themselves in. As such, Billig (1996) argues that the stock of ideas and ways of thinking that surround an object – like PrEP – will always be riddled with controversy or contradictions. Moscovici and Marková (2000: p 275) argue that, as a result, social representations inevitably involve an ongoing 'battle of ideas', which makes them inherently dynamic and dilemmatic. These diverging and opposing views and ideas are 'in the world', but also enter our 'head' (Farr, 1987: p 359). This creates a complex reality for both individuals and communities – a reality in which PrEP has seemingly contradictory and paradoxical qualities that, however, can all be considered true. Within SRT, this has been referred to as cognitive polyphasia. Jovchelovitch (2007: p 69) defines cognitive polyphasia as 'a state in which different kinds of knowledge, possessing different rationalities, live side by side in the same individual or collective'. This not only opens up an avenue towards an understanding of how opposing ideas can coexist, but also enables me to explore how individuals and communities encounter and respond to opposing ideas through what I term 'everyday PrEP negotiations' (see Box 1.1 for a definition). It is through everyday PrEP negotiations that some social representations achieve greater legitimacy, or influence on people's engagement with PrEP, even when other views are recognised.

> **Box 1.1: Definition of 'everyday PrEP negotiations'**
>
> Everyday PrEP negotiations are the continuous and often subtle mental activities and social interactions that individuals engage in within a particular context to understand, interpret, and navigate the opposing and contradictory ideas and ways of thinking about PrEP that they encounter in daily life. This includes all the deliberations, reflections, and sense-making activities that people continuously engage in to give meaning to PrEP and its role in their lives. It also includes the day-to-day interactions in which people discuss shared experiences, reflect on, challenge, or further bolster certain ideas, practices, or norms about PrEP.

Cognitive polyphasia does not automatically consider contradictory ways of thinking and what we can call the 'battle of ideas' to be problematic, although of course they can be. While contention, uncertainty, dilemmas, and ambiguity may, on the face of it, seem unproductive, Billig (1996) and Marková (1987) argue that the battle of ideas within people and in society can be productive in triggering thought and reflection, with counter-ideas deepening knowledge of, commitment to, and sense-making of certain values, ideas, and practices. Recognising how opposing and contradictory ideas and ways of thinking can trigger everyday PrEP negotiations that may be more or less productive is critical to informing initiatives that make PrEP 'work for' more people.

Figure 1.1 attempts to visually summarise the previous discussion in a Venn diagram. It captures the fact that there are opposing and contradictory ideas out there 'in the world', with some appearing as contrary to (*para* in Greek) held opinion (*doxa* in Greek). These contrary ideas exist in society, circulate within communities, and make their entry 'in the head'. They can trigger a battle of ideas leading to contention, uncertainty, dilemmas, and ambiguity. In the process, people may find themselves in a liminal state where, through everyday PrEP negotiations, they weigh up and balance the legitimacy and influence of different ideas.

The conceptual framework presented in Figure 1.1 was not developed a priori but constructed in close dialogue with my

Figure 1.1: The social representations paradox model

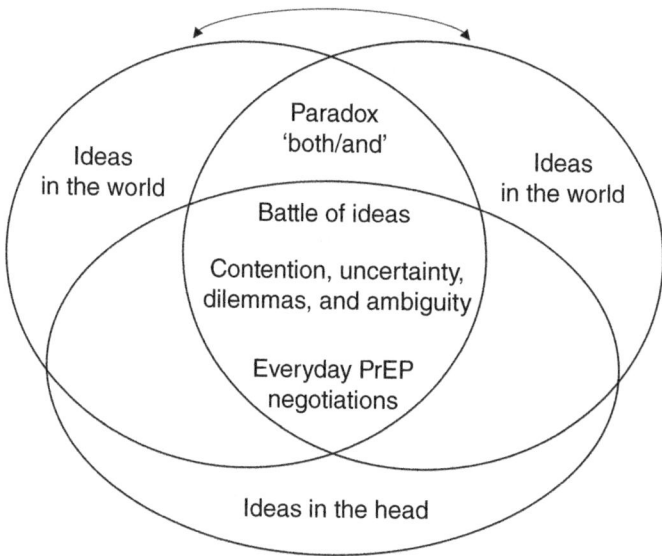

data. I therefore hope that readers can see alignment between the framework and the findings presented. The empirical chapters will each focus on a PrEP paradox. These PrEP paradox chapters are each divided into three sections, each of which details an everyday PrEP negotiation and follows the structure outlined in Table 2.3. Their headings first present an interpretively constructed question that alludes to contention, uncertainty, dilemmas, and ambiguity. The question is followed by a type of everyday PrEP negotiation work. It is my hope that if people taking, or interested in, PrEP read this book, they will identify with many of the questions and find comfort in the recognition of their everyday PrEP negotiation work. As I elaborate on the everyday PrEP negotiations, I detail the stock of ideas and ways of thinking that are at play, and emphasise how social context mediates how people encounter, respond to, and negotiate PrEP use.

Introducing the chapters and paradoxes covered in this book

Following this Introduction, Chapter 2 describes our research with adolescent girls and young women in Zimbabwe and with queer men in Denmark. I describe the two studies in turn, detailing and reflecting upon the fieldwork and methods applied. I end Chapter 2 by discussing the opportunities and challenges of generating learning from two very different case studies.

Chapter 3 introduces the first paradox covered in this book: *Free, yet costly*. This chapter notes that although PrEP is recognised as free from clinics in both study settings, it is also associated with costs. This chapter details what those costs are and exemplifies how our participants negotiate ideas about these costs in everyday life.

Chapter 4 introduces the second paradox: *Eligible, yet ineligible*. The chapter finds that although many of our study participants consider themselves eligible for PrEP, they also have their eligibility challenged by others. This chapter focuses on demonstrating how people taking, or interested in, PrEP navigate such different ideas and negotiate their eligibility.

Chapter 5 introduces the third paradox: *Responsible, yet irresponsible*. This chapter focuses almost exclusively on queer men. It reports on how queer PrEP users may be considered responsible for taking control over their sexual health and for contributing to the prevention of HIV response, yet at the same are confronted with ideas about their irresponsible sexual behaviour.

Chapter 6 introduces the fourth paradox, which is the paradox I alluded to in the opening of the book: *Healthy, yet a patient*. This chapter details how, for people on PrEP, the close contact with health services and daily pill-taking are constant reminders of how their sexuality is being pathologised and approached like a disease requiring treatment. Some PrEP users struggle to reconcile this pathologising, and the treatment regimen, with being healthy.

Chapter 7 covers the fifth paradox: *Safe, yet unsafe*. This chapter finds that while PrEP users fully recognise the potential of PrEP to keep them safe from contracting HIV, they have to balance this protective capacity against opposing ideas about PrEP's associations with social risks and harms.

Chapter 8 introduces the sixth and final paradox: *Liberating, yet constraining*. This chapter covers ambiguities related to the sexual liberation associated with PrEP. PrEP users in both contexts express a newly found sexual freedom when on PrEP. PrEP is said to remove feelings of fear of HIV and to give PrEP users a sense of control and autonomy over their sexuality. Alongside this sense of liberation are feelings of constraint. These feelings manifest differently from person to person. For some, the treatment regimen – having to take a daily pill and attend regular health checks – puts constraints on their daily life. For others, the liberating effects of PrEP can be addictive and they find it challenging to stop being on PrEP, even if they are no longer vulnerable to HIV.

Chapters 3–8 are empirical chapters and introduce data from the two studies. The chapters are presented in such a way that they capture the paradoxes along the HIV prevention cascade, covering the effects of PrEP paradoxes on motivation for PrEP use, access, and sustained use (Moorhouse et al., 2019). By structuring the book according to the paradoxes, I run the risk of hiding the connections between the paradoxes. While I will do my best to signpost potential connections, I kindly ask you, as a reader, to make mental notes whenever you see one. Chapter 9 concludes the book by discussing a possible seventh paradox, namely that PrEP paradoxes are *problematic, yet productive*.

TWO

The case studies

This book draws on qualitative research conducted in Zimbabwe and Denmark with people taking, interested in, or eligible for PrEP. Both studies had an applied interest to increase uptake of PrEP, and sought to produce knowledge that can be used by HIV prevention service planners and practitioners to improve PrEP uptake and utilisation. Stakeholder involvement was a guiding principle of both studies. As such, both studies were striving to do the research 'with' and 'by' people either taking or interested in PrEP, and not merely 'about' or 'for' them. This chapter provides a reflexive account of the research process. This involves first reflecting on my stance on and approach to the topic of PrEP. I then provide some background to the two case studies and contexts, and use this to explain my comparative focus. I then describe the research processes. I here explain the methods used, how participants were recruited, and how data were produced and prepared for analysis. I end the chapter by explaining how data were examined for the analyses presented in subsequent chapters.

Reflexivity and power

In alignment with many feminist and critical social researchers, I am acutely aware that there is no value-free scientific inquiry, and that researchers must 'acknowledge their interests and sympathies' (Ellis et al., 1997: p 123). To that end, I proclaim that the methodologies guiding the two case studies of this book have been steered by community health psychology, a subdiscipline 'driven by values of power-sharing and social justice, and [that] is praxis-oriented, emphasising solidarity with oppressed people to create transformative social change' (Nelson and Evans, 2014: p 158). This interest, coupled with the fact that I am a Caucasian and privileged researcher working in the field of global health, based at a renowned university in Denmark, has heightened my awareness of power inequalities, and my role as a researcher in reproducing them. Participatory methodologies offer one way to support shifts away from Global North researchers 'having power' to 'sharing power', which hopefully one day will lead to a 'handover of power'. While I actively use participatory approaches and methods aimed at giving participants more power and control over how their lived realities are represented, and strive to co-write with participants in book chapters and articles, in *this* writing project I acknowledge my limits in this participatory endeavour and further acknowledge my role in reproducing power inequalities. However, I hope that by inviting a few participants to review and comment on earlier drafts of this book, I have succeeded in making the book resonate with their experiences of PrEP. Nonetheless, this book is solo-authored, and I inevitably take credit for work and ideas that are the result of many conversations with colleagues and our collective efforts (please see my acknowledgements in the Preface).

Having said that, I am not merely a privileged outsider. I too constitute a stakeholder in PrEP research. I am part of the 'us' in the slogan 'nothing about us, without us', which has guided much HIV research and practice. As a queer man, the devastating effect of HIV is a heritage of my community. Fear and the stigma of HIV has had a profound effect on my sexuality and that of my friends and peers. I have personally witnessed and experienced the impacts and effects of HIV and PrEP on people's lives. This background inevitably affects how I frame and analyse the data, and the conclusions I draw.

Introducing the Zimbabwean context and case study

The Zimbabwean case study focuses on adolescent girls and young women vulnerable to HIV. Gender and other inequalities leave adolescent girls and young women in sub-Saharan Africa at particularly high risk of HIV infection. In 2022, women and girls accounted for 63 per cent of all new infections on the African continent (UNAIDS, 2023), a pattern that is no different in Zimbabwe. In Zimbabwe the HIV prevalence for men aged 25–29 is 4 per cent, whereas the HIV prevalence for women in the same age group is 10.6 per cent (Ministry of Health and Child Care, 2021). Given this inequity, the Joint United Nations Programme on HIV/AIDS has made repeated calls for research and action to make PrEP more accessible to girls and women.

Against this background, and with support from international donors, expanding the roll-out of free PrEP for young women is a priority area of the Zimbabwe National HIV and AIDS Strategic Plan (Ministry of Health and Child Care & National AIDS Council, 2020). See Table 2.1 for a summary of PrEP services in Zimbabwe. While great strides have been made to reach female sex workers with PrEP in Zimbabwe (Matambanadzo et al., 2021), progress to reach adolescent girls and young women with an elevated chance of contracting HIV has been slow.

In light of this, we initiated the Youth of Zimbabwe Use HIV Prevention (YZ-UHP) study in 2017, a randomised trial and intervention study designed to explore the impact of tablet-based education and counselling, combined with community engagement, on improving uptake and use of condoms, PrEP, and voluntary male circumcision among young people in Manicaland province, eastern Zimbabwe (Thomas et al., 2020a, 2020b). It is a mixed-methods study, and as a co-investigator and community health psychologist, I facilitated the qualitative research and the community engagement intervention aimed at improving the uptake and use of HIV prevention methods.

The Zimbabwe data presented in this book come from the YZ-UHP study. The study was designed with a commitment to participatory research practice. First, a youth advisory board was established to advise us on the different phases of the project. Second, community interventions were co-created through community conversations, resulting in different community-led initiatives. Third, the qualitative work was extensive, and, in addition to interviews and focus group discussions, drew on Photovoice, a visual methodology that allows participants to photographically capture and represent issues of importance to them. The YZ-UHP study obtained ethical approvals from the Medical Research Council of Zimbabwe (REF: MRCZ/A/2243), the institutional review board of the Biomedical Research and Training Institute in Zimbabwe (REF: AP140/2017), and the Imperial College London Research Ethics Committee (REF: 17IC4160).

In this book I draw on qualitative work with presumably straight adolescent and young women from two communities, which we refer to as Watku and Saksom. Watku is a rural community, while Saksom is a high-density suburban community. Both communities are located in Manicaland, a province that borders Mozambique. The province is the second most populous province of Zimbabwe, with just over 2 million people (Zimbabwe National Statistics Agency, 2022). The province is characterised by high levels of poverty. About two-thirds of people who live in Manicaland struggle with absolute poverty. The formal sector is small, and most people rely on subsistence farming and government or donor assistance. With a declining, yet still high, HIV prevalence of 12.3 per cent for women and 9.8 per cent for men, HIV continues to be a major challenge for the people of Manicaland, particularly for young women aged 20–24, where the gender disparity is the largest (Rao et al., 2022). Age-disparate relationships are common in

Manicaland (Chang et al., 2021), and HIV incidence rates are particularly high among girls in relationships with older men (Schaefer et al., 2017).

The vulnerabilities faced by many young women stem from certain cultural gender norms. These norms deserve discussion and provide critical context for some of the findings presented in this book.

The Shona people are the largest ethnic group in Manicaland. Patriarchal practices are rife in Shona culture, with hegemonic forms of masculinity still subjecting many women to subordination – perpetuating gender inequalities as outlined earlier. Kambarami (2006) notes that in Shona culture boys and girls are socialised very differently. Her research finds that girls are socialised to become submissive and obedient wives and caring mothers, whereas boys are socialised to become heads of the household. Boys and girls also often have their sexuality defined for them. Girls are expected to preserve their virginity for marriage, with *mombe yechimanda* – a cultural practice of offering a cow to the girl's parents as a token of appreciation for preserving her virginity – still holding much value (Matswetu and Bhana, 2018). In marriage, a woman is expected to remain faithful and to be submissive to the sexual needs of her husband. In contrast, boys and young men are taught that they must control female sexuality and that male infidelity is inevitable. Such patriarchal socialisation practices in Zimbabwean society shape how men and women relate to each other in all areas of life, leaving young women especially vulnerable to intimate partner violence (Fidan and Bui, 2016) and HIV, as previously described. Many women in Zimbabwe are thus always in a gendered and dyadic relationship with men. Several studies from Zimbabwe demonstrate that women's actions and engagement with HIV treatment and prevention services must always be considered against a background of how men relate to women (Skovdal et al., 2011; Chibango and Potgieter, 2023). The impact of patriarchy and the dyadic relationship between men and women on young women's engagement with PrEP will become clear as I present our findings. While patriarchy and hegemonic masculinities dominate and constitute a critical context for the Zimbabwe case, I also want to recognise that patriarchal practices undergo constant negotiation, translation, and reconfiguration (Demetriou, 2001). A few of the young women participating in our study exemplify this by expressing support and care from their husbands.

Much qualitative material from the YZ-UHP study has already been published, highlighting several social challenges to young women's engagement with PrEP. These challenges include stigma and breaches of confidentiality by healthcare providers (Skovdal et al., 2021), parental disapproval of young women's premarital and extramarital sexual activities (Skovdal et al., 2023), and the perceived social risks associated with partners finding out about young women's potential PrEP use (Skovdal et al., 2022a). Additionally, the lack of community-level awareness about PrEP and its benefits has been identified as a contributing factor (Skovdal et al., 2022b). This book expands on some of these findings, albeit with a focus on how social circumstances shape the paradoxical ideas and ways of thinking that surround PrEP and affect the work involved with PrEP use.

Introducing the Danish context and case study

The Danish case study focuses on queer men vulnerable to HIV. As in many other European countries, gay, bisexual, and other queer men who have sex with men in Denmark are disproportionately affected by HIV and constitute the main target group of PrEP. According to the Statens Serum Institut, a research institute working under the auspices of the Ministry of Health in Denmark, an estimated 6,300 individuals lived with HIV in Denmark in 2022 (SSI, 2023). More than half of those (3,500) were queer men. Of 115 newly diagnosed HIV positives in 2022, 47 were among queer men.

PrEP was approved and recommended by the Danish Health Authority in 2017 and made freely available through the national health services in 2019. The fact that PrEP is made available cost-free is unusual for a couple of reasons. First, although Denmark has a universal and tax-financed national health service, there are two primary exclusions to its coverage, including outpatient prescription drugs and adult dental care, both of which require co-payment (Birk et al., 2024). Second, the Danish healthcare system has a far greater focus on curative care, with only few resources allocated to health promotion and disease prevention (Birk et al., 2024). Health promotion activities are often non-medical and fall under the auspices of municipalities or non-governmental organisations. The exclusion of a co-payment for a preventive and outpatient drug like PrEP makes it stand out and subject to controversy. As such, the roll-out of PrEP in Denmark – like in the UK – did not happen without contention and public debate, much of which was rooted in the assumed immorality of 'unsafe' and 'promiscuous' sex between gay men. For instance, both health economists, a member of the Danish Council on Ethics as well as politicians have called for gay men to take individual responsibility by paying for the pills themselves, using condoms, or reducing so-called risky behaviours (TV2, 2016; BT, 2016).

One other feature of PrEP provision in Denmark stands out and deserves mentioning. PrEP can only be accessed through hospitals with infectious disease departments. Prescriptions and the distribution of PrEP can only be made by medical doctors specialising in infectious diseases. As such, individuals interested in PrEP must be referred to one of nine infectious disease departments either by their general practitioner or by Checkpoint, a chain of queer-friendly sexual health clinics spread out across major cities in Denmark. See Table 2.1 for a summary of PrEP services in Denmark.

PrEP has proved popular in the queer community. In its first year, 1,180 individuals were put on PrEP. This number increased to 1,500 in 2021 and 2,000 in 2022. By 1 September 2023, 3,998 individuals had started on PrEP, of whom 3,385 were registered as active users (Engsig and Kronborg, 2024). The investment in PrEP is paying off, as it has proven effective in Denmark. Since the 1990s, new HIV cases among queer men have averaged around 75 annually, but following the introduction of PrEP, newly diagnosed HIV cases have more than halved to 29 cases in 2023 (Nielsen, 2023).

The Danish case study draws on qualitative data from what we can refer to as the 'PrEPping project', a community-based participatory research project that was initiated in 2021 with funding from AIDS-Fondet. AIDS-Fondet is a Danish non-governmental organisation that provides sexual health counselling and testing services and supports research and advocacy. The project aimed to develop a knowledge foundation for delivering PrEP services in Denmark that are relevant and acceptable for individuals at elevated risk of HIV. Community-based participatory research is a collaborative research approach whereby community members, stakeholders, and researchers work together through co-research to understand and address issues and concerns that are relevant and meaningful to the community under study (Minkler and Wallerstein, 2003). The study team was made up of two queer men with PrEP experience, two PrEP service providers, and two academic researchers – a research assistant and me. Specific study aims and research tools were co-created by the study team and centred on queer men's experiences of considering, accessing, and being on PrEP. This project also drew on the Photovoice methodology, enabling queer men to share their stories, experiences, and perspectives through images. The project was registered and approved from a data protection perspective by a University of Copenhagen faculty secretariat and received approval from a university ethics review committee (REF: 504-0256/21-5000).

A comparative case study

My two cases differ markedly from each other. They took place in countries with vastly different experiences of the HIV epidemic. In Zimbabwe, HIV is endemic and generalised. Everyone has been affected one way or another. In Denmark, HIV is close to being eliminated and largely limited to a few population groups vulnerable to it. This country-specific information leads to a natural focus on groups most vulnerable to HIV, namely young straight women in Zimbabwe and queer men in Denmark.

The differing HIV epidemiologies of the two countries have affected their HIV service landscape. Zimbabwe is decentralising PrEP services to increase access to anyone who considers themselves to be vulnerable to HIV, whereas PrEP services in Denmark are highly centralised and focused on individuals who meet predefined and strict eligibility criteria. Table 2.1 offers a comparative overview of PrEP services in the two countries.

Other major differences between the two countries are their respective economies and social welfare contexts. The Denmark case is an example of a rich, modern welfare state with social insurance contributing to healthcare and other social benefits. Given the large informal economy of Zimbabwe, social protection arrangements are patchy and user-fee payments for hospital services are relatively common. However, HIV services in Zimbabwe are free, part-funded by the Ministry of Health and Child Care, with contributions also from international organisations.

This brings me to some of the similarities between Denmark and Zimbabwe. PrEP is freely available in both countries and was made available more or less at the same time. This reflects their shared commitment to the HIV response, which is also captured in their successes in getting people living with HIV onto treatment. Both countries rank highly in terms of achieving the 95–95–95 goals referred to in the Introduction (UNAIDS, 2023).

Much in-depth qualitative research on PrEP focuses on experiences in single-country contexts or from the perspective of a single target group. Such important work provides detailed case studies of how PrEP is delivered and experienced in

Table 2.1: PrEP services in Zimbabwe and Denmark

Oral PrEP services	Zimbabwe	Denmark
Roll-out	Started in 2018, but still ongoing	2019
Cost for users	Free, state- and international donor-funded	Free, state-funded
Target groups	Anyone with an increased chance of contracting HIV	Men or transgender individuals who have sex with men
Criteria to qualify	• HIV negative • Member of target group • Normal kidney function • Agree to and follow treatment guidelines	• HIV negative • Member of target group • 15 years or older • Increased chance of contracting HIV • Normal kidney function • Agree to and follow treatment guidelines • Danish social security number • Heterosexual individuals with elevated risk of HIV may also be eligible
How 'increased chance of contracting HIV' is assessed	Belong to one of the following groups: • Serodiscordant couples (one HIV-negative partner) • Adolescent girls and young women • Sex workers • Certain groups of men (men who have sex with men, prisoners, long-distance truck drivers) • Transgender people • Anyone with a history of condomless anal sex,	At least one of the following criteria must be met: • Having had unprotected anal intercourse with at least two male partners within the last 12 weeks • Having contracted syphilis, chlamydia, or gonorrhea within the last 24 weeks

(continued)

Table 2.1: PrEP services in Zimbabwe and Denmark (continued)

Oral PrEP services	Zimbabwe	Denmark
	having had a sexually transmitted infection, has a sexual partner who is vulnerable to HIV, or past use of post-exposure prophylaxis	
PrEP service package	*PrEP initiation* • PrEP eligibility assessment • Testing for HIV, sexually transmitted infections, and kidney function (age dependent) • Assessment of pregnancy status • 1-month PrEP prescription *PrEP follow-up/continuation* • Month 1 (review side effects and give 2-month PrEP refill) • Month 3 (controls as at initiation and PrEP refills every 3 months)	*PrEP initiation* • PrEP eligibility assessment • Testing for HIV, sexually transmitted infections, and kidney function • 3-month PrEP prescription • Counselling on safe sex practices *PrEP follow-up/continuation* • Month 3 (controls as at initiation and PrEP refills every 3–6 months)
PrEP service locations	Hospitals, clinics, and other settings where HIV testing is done	Nine hospital-based infectious disease clinics and through Checkpoint, a queer-friendly and designated sexual health clinic in five major cities
PrEP service providers	Doctors, nurses, and HIV testing counsellors	Infectious disease doctors and nurses
PrEP service frequency	PrEP initiation same day as HIV-negative test or within 7 days, Months 1 and 3 follow-ups, every 3 months thereafter	Health facility visits every 3–6 months after initiation

different contexts, and responds to calls for research that looks at sexual health interventions in context (Wellings et al., 2006). Important as this is, such work is often blind to issues that cut across population and country contexts, and thus fall short of developing generalisable lessons and concepts; this, however, is possible through comparative case studies (Yin, 2003). There have generally been few comparative studies of PrEP in the 'mixed economy of welfare' (Powell, 2019). By bringing together and comparing two such different cases, I apply what Schensul et al. (1999) call a 'dichotomous case selection'. This heightens my attention to factors that may explain differences and similarities. Nicolini (2009) argues that there are benefits to looking at practices (such as PrEP use) in different settings, repositioning oneself by 'zooming in' to understand the situated performance of, for instance, PrEP use, and 'zooming out' to see broader relations, patterns, and effects across different localities. In this book I both zoom in on people's experiences of PrEP in Zimbabwe and Denmark, and zoom out to conceptually highlight fundamental paradoxes and the type of work they necessitate. In doing so, I hope to create some productive and novel cross-cultural comparisons.

It is important to highlight that the two studies I draw on in this book were not conducted for the purpose of a comparative case study analysis. As such, the research tools were not deliberately streamlined to investigate similar issues. Nonetheless, given that my involvement and input into both studies affected the issues covered and the choice of qualitative methods, there are many similarities between the two data sets. I now describe these similarities in more detail.

The research process

Individual interviews and Photovoice were the two primary methods used to gain an in-depth understanding of the experiences and perspectives of individuals either taking or interested in PrEP. Three focus group discussions were also conducted in Zimbabwe. This is the material I directly draw on this analysis. I also have interview material from healthcare providers in both settings, and material from parents, partners, and community members in Zimbabwe; while I will not introduce this material in this book, it has corroborated and enriched my thinking about and analysis of the paradoxes. Furthermore, I live in Denmark as a member of the queer community, know people on PrEP, and have conducted HIV research in Zimbabwe since 2010, which all contributes to the lived experience and observational 'data' that I bring to the analysis.

Various strategies were employed to recruit individuals either taking or eligible for PrEP. For the YZ-UHP study in Zimbabwe, young women eligible for PrEP were randomly sampled from a baseline survey in which they had to fulfil criteria such as being young, HIV negative, sexually active, and with an increased likelihood of contracting HIV. The women on PrEP were recruited from a follow-up survey that captured PrEP use. All the young women had previously given permission for, and expressed interest in, being contacted to participate in qualitative research. The PrEPping project in Denmark adopted different recruitment strategies, taking advantage of the diversity within the study team. The two queer co-researchers shared details about the study within their social network, and the two PrEP providers shared information about the study with their clients. The researchers put up posters in different venues and on Facebook pages and made use of a paid advertisement on Instagram. These different strategies resulted in the recruitment of 39 young women in Zimbabwe and 16 queer men in Denmark. See Table 2.2 for participant characteristics.

In both cases, the data collection process started with Photovoice, a method that involves inviting study participants to photographically capture and represent issues of importance to them (Wang and Burris, 1997). In the YZ-UHP study, Photovoice was, for practical reasons, limited to

Table 2.2: Study participant characteristics

Zimbabwe		
Rural/urban residence	Rural (Watku)	17
	Urban (Saksom)	22
Gender	Cis female	39
Age	18–24	25
	25+	5
	Undeclared	9
Country of origin	Zimbabwe (Shona ethnic group)	39
PrEP status	Eligible for PrEP	19
	On PrEP	6
	Undeclared	14
Denmark		
Rural/urban residence	Rural	0
	Urban	16
Gender	Cis male	14
	Gender-fluid male	1
	Trans man	1
Age	18–24	2
	25–34	7
	35+	7
Country of origin	Canada	1
	China	1
	Denmark	10
	Greenland	1
	Slovakia	1
	Sweden	1
	Venezuela	1
PrEP status	Eligible for PrEP	3
	Former PrEP user, wants to start again	1
	On PrEP	12

five individuals: adolescent girls and young women. While all 16 queer men in the PrEPping project were invited to participate in Photovoice, only 13 participants completed the exercise.

Photovoice participants in both settings were introduced to the method and exercise through a workshop, where the research aims were fine-tuned to reflect the interests of the participants; ethical considerations were also discussed. The young women in Zimbabwe were given disposable cameras, while the queer men in Denmark used their smartphones; consequently, the quality of the images in the book is varied, and due to permissions issues, details in some images have been blurred. The participants were given two to three weeks to photograph things, places, and people that affect their experiences and perceptions of and access to PrEP. Photovoice participants in both settings were invited to select up to six photographs that represented a story they really wanted to tell in relation to PrEP, and that they were willing both to share with the public through exhibitions and to hand over to the research teams as data for publications. They were encouraged to write a story for each of their chosen photographs, explaining why they wanted to share this picture, the real story behind it, and how it related to their life and the lives of other people. The exercise resulted in 76 photographs from queer men in Denmark and 36 photographs from young women in Zimbabwe, each accompanied by a written story. The Photovoice exercise in Denmark culminated in a photo exhibition during the 2022 Copenhagen Pride week (see Figure 2.1).

Photovoice was followed by individual interviews designed to elicit detailed experiences and perceptions of PrEP. The interviews in both settings were semi-structured and followed topic guides that focused on the participants' knowledge of and motivation for using PrEP, the role of social relations, attitudes, and practices in shaping their PrEP use, their perspectives on PrEP services, and what PrEP can offer them, as either young

Figure 2.1: 'Picturing PrEP' exhibition

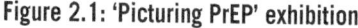

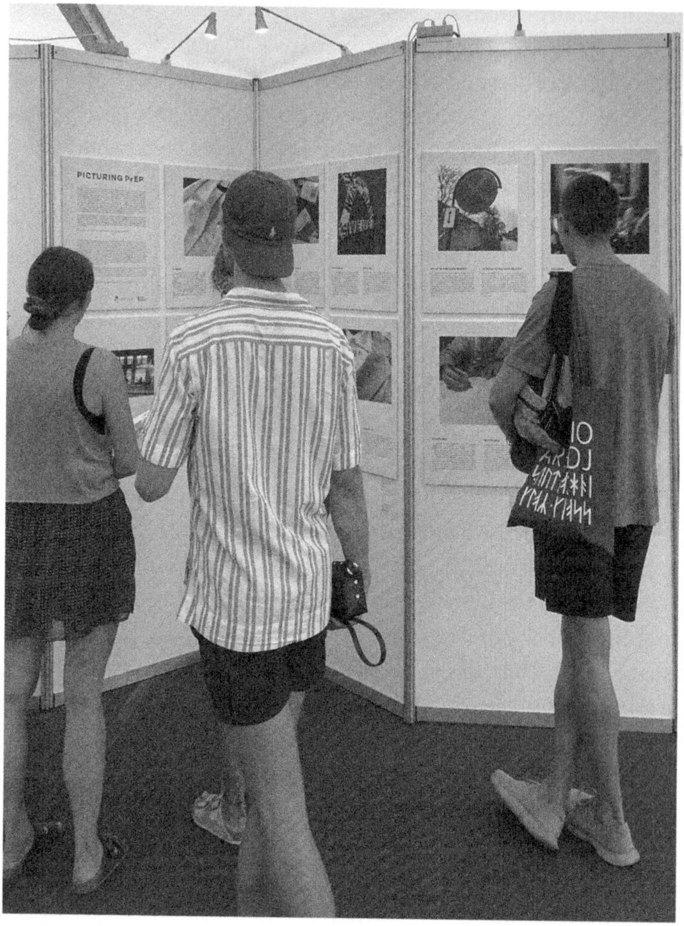

women or queer men. Where interviewees had participated in Photovoice, the six photographs that represented a story they really wanted to tell were also discussed. All interviewees contextualised PrEP in relation to their lived experiences of being either young women or queer men. However, interviews with PrEP users maintained a focus on lived experiences, whereas with individuals eligible for PrEP, topics on PrEP use naturally focused more on their beliefs, perspectives, and anecdotal or 'hearsay' information. The interviews were digitally recorded and chiefly conducted in Shona (Zimbabwe case) or Danish (Denmark case). As four of the queer men were not fluent in Danish, their interviews were conducted in English. Interviews with the queer men lasted on average 56 minutes, whereas interviews with the young women took an average of 50 minutes.

The research methods described earlier were implemented by trained and highly experienced qualitative researchers. The research activities with young women in Zimbabwe were facilitated by Rangarirayi Primrose Nyamwanza, a young woman who is trained and has worked as a social worker. This background made her particularly well suited for in-depth discussions on sexuality, gender, and some of the more taboo and controversial aspects of these topics. She gained the trust of the female participants and connected with them due to their shared identities and gender experiences, making her a peer researcher (Primdahl et al., 2021). The 'sisterhood' that developed between Nyamwanza and the young women in our study inevitably helped develop and shape the data.

The research activities with queer men in Denmark were also facilitated by a young woman: Nina Langer Primdahl. As a straight, cisgender woman, she did not share the same gender and sexual identity as the queer men. However, as a seasoned researcher of sexual minorities, she was able to build rapport with the participants and was well versed in the language and culture of queer men. As the transcripts and data presented in this book demonstrate, the queer men felt they could speak freely and without judgement.

All interviews were transcribed and anonymised. They were, together with Photovoice pictures and stories, imported into NVivo 14, a computer-assisted qualitative analysis software. From here, four master's students (Clausen, Sørensen,

Quistgaard, and Vyas), a research assistant (Primdahl), the queer men (Hanghøj and 'José') and PrEP service providers (Borchmann, Vincentz) who formed part of the study team in Denmark, three collaborators in Zimbabwe (Nyamukapa, Magoge-Mandizvidza, and Maswera), and I interrogated the data from different vantage points, guided by and responding to different research questions. We have reported or will be reporting on these findings and the analytical processes elsewhere (Skovdal et al., 2021; Primdahl et al., 2022; Skovdal et al., 2022a; Primdahl and Skovdal, 2023). Through these collaborative analyses (Cornish et al., 2013), researchers with diverse expertise – including social workers, medical professionals, and community advocates with lived experience of PrEP – came together to highlight different aspects of PrEP use. Combined with our participatory research approach, this process helped to unveil the paradoxes rooted in lived experiences and practice. As I participated in these collaborative analyses, it became clear to me that six paradoxes feature prominently in people's experiences of PrEP, irrespective of whether they are queer men in Denmark or young women living in Zimbabwe. To zoom in on these paradoxes, two student assistants (Biermann and Hansen) and I followed Attride-Stirling's (2001) steps of thematic network analysis to reorganise and code the data. This resulted in six thematic networks, each detailing the content and context of a PrEP paradox. In close dialogue with Biermann and the social representations paradox model (see Figure 1.1), I condensed and further reorganised the networks into a single table (see Table 2.3). The table captures the connections between the paradoxes, everyday PrEP negotiations, the opposing ideas and ways of thinking at play, and the mediating role of social context. In subsequent chapters I draw on this table to structure and present findings.

Table 2.3: Thematic network table of findings

Paradoxes	Everyday PrEP negotiations	Opposing ideas and 'ways of thinking' that give rise to contention, uncertainty, dilemmas, and ambiguity	Social context of ideas and 'ways of thinking' that mediate and amplify everyday PrEP negotiations
Free, yet costly (PrEP is free in both contexts, yet associated with costs)	Why do I have free access? *Making sense* of privileged access to costly PrEP	• Inequalities in access due to high drug prices foster recognition of privilege (Z, DK) • Public controversy surrounding free PrEP pushes queer men to account for their privilege (DK) • Accountability to past activist work (DK)	• Media discourses • Historic marginalisation • Responsibilisation within a social welfare system
	Is it really free? *Balancing* out-of-pocket expenses with HIV vulnerabilities	• It costs money to travel and reach free PrEP services (Z) • Hospital fees are expected when accessing free PrEP (Z) • Poverty as a barrier to young women's access to free PrEP (Z)	• Health system financing • Poverty and conditions of living • Women's reliance on men
	Is free PrEP worth it? *Thinking critically* about PrEP service delivery	• PrEP services are costly in terms of time spent accessing PrEP (DK) • Free PrEP services are inaccessible due to high opportunity costs (Z)	• Rigid and centralised PrEP services • Poverty and conditions of living • Women's reliance on men

Table 2.3: Thematic network table of findings (continued)

Paradoxes	Everyday PrEP negotiations	Opposing ideas and 'ways of thinking' that give rise to contention, uncertainty, dilemmas, and ambiguity	Social context of ideas and 'ways of thinking' that mediate and amplify everyday PrEP negotiations
Eligible, yet ineligible (People may be eligible for PrEP, yet have their eligibility challenged)	Are 'good girls' on PrEP? *Considering* cultural eligibility criteria	• Parents or other guardians often disapprove of PrEP use (Z) • Partners often disapprove of PrEP use (Z)	• Traditional understandings of young women's sexuality • 'Good girl' notions
	How will others view my eligibility? *Fearing* stigmatising associations with PrEP use	• PrEP was initially introduced to, and is still considered an HIV prevention method for, sex workers (Z) • HIV stigma and secrecy feed ideas about PrEP as a cover-up for antiretroviral therapy (Z)	• PrEP initially introduced to sex workers • PrEP delivered through HIV services
	Should I lie or appeal for eligibility? *Navigating* 'the system' and *negotiating* eligibility	• Eligibility talked about as a chicken-and-egg situation (DK) • Lying about eligibility is considered a prerequisite for access and to reap the broad benefits of PrEP (DK) • Appealing for PrEP services to deliver personalised care (Z)	• Biopolitical and resource-related restrictions on who qualifies for PrEP • Rigidity of 'the system' and who qualifies for eligibility

(continued)

Table 2.3: Thematic network table of findings (continued)

Paradoxes	Everyday PrEP negotiations	Opposing ideas and 'ways of thinking' that give rise to contention, uncertainty, dilemmas, and ambiguity	Social context of ideas and 'ways of thinking' that mediate and amplify everyday PrEP negotiations
Responsible, yet irresponsible (People on PrEP take responsibility for their sexual health, yet are confronted with negative ideas about their irresponsible sexual behaviours)	Am I taking responsibility for my sexual health? *Negotiating* 'PrEP responsibility' in a relational context	• Negotiating condom use in the 'heat of the moment' is challenging, making PrEP a responsible thing to do (DK, Z) • PrEP as a license for 'irresponsible' condomless anal sex (DK) • PrEP and condomless anal sex are associated with increases in (more drug-resistant) sexually transmitted infections (DK)	• Representation of PrEP users as vectors of sexually transmitted infections • Grindr amplifies different (ir)responsibilities • (Ir)responsibilities are talked about differently in social networks
	Why do I feel irresponsible when taking responsibility? *Shame* associated with PrEP	• PrEP signals promiscuity and past 'irresponsible' behaviour (DK) • Condomless anal sex is considered irresponsible and shameful (DK)	• (Self-)stigma surrounding queer sex • PrEP services and eligibility criteria accentuate past 'irresponsible' sexual behaviours • Social networks reframe 'sayings'
	Am *I* irresponsible? 'Othering' non-PrEP users	• Non-PrEP users are talked about as boring, traditional, and irresponsible (DK) • PrEP users have certain qualities and the strength to be different (Z)	• Social networks enable favourable biases and positive social identities around PrEP use

Table 2.3: Thematic network table of findings (continued)

Paradoxes	Everyday PrEP negotiations	Opposing ideas and 'ways of thinking' that give rise to contention, uncertainty, dilemmas, and ambiguity	Social context of ideas and 'ways of thinking' that mediate and amplify everyday PrEP negotiations
Healthy, yet a patient (People on PrEP are healthy, yet required to adopt a 'patient' persona)	What am I treating when I am not sick? *Difficulties reconciling* the 'patient' persona with being healthy	• Taking pills for prevention is considered nonsensical (Z) • Taking pills for prevention is considered overwhelming (DK)	• Dissonance between pill-taking and being healthy • The hospitalisation of PrEP services in Denmark pathologises the issue
	How do I give meaning to PrEP treatment? *Rethinking* PrEP as a treatment to maintain health	• Rejecting the pathologising of PrEP (DK) • PrEP is rationalised as self-care and part of a healthy lifestyle (DK, Z)	• PrEP considered key by young women to prevent them contracting HIV from unfaithful partners • PrEP signals taking control of and responsibility for maintaining good health
	Is it worth it? *Weighing up* the preventive potential against side effects and HIV	• Anticipated side effects prevent engagement with PrEP and may outweigh risk perception (Z) • Uncertainty about the value of taking a preventive pill in the context of antiretroviral therapy (Z, DK)	• Collective memory of side effects related to antiretroviral drugs • Improvements in antiretroviral treatment make HIV less intimidating • Limited PrEP awareness

(continued)

Table 2.3: Thematic network table of findings (continued)

Paradoxes	Everyday PrEP negotiations	Opposing ideas and 'ways of thinking' that give rise to contention, uncertainty, dilemmas, and ambiguity	Social context of ideas and 'ways of thinking' that mediate and amplify everyday PrEP negotiations
Safe, yet unsafe (PrEP keeps people safe from contracting HIV, yet is associated with other risks and harm)	What social risks come with PrEP? *Weighing up* the perceived dangers against protection against HIV	• Widespread shared understanding of the lack of social acceptability of PrEP (Z) • PrEP keeps you safe from HIV, but when taken discreetly, and if discovered, may lead to domestic violence (Z) • You may disappoint parents or partners, leading to risk of abandonment (Z)	• Patriarchy and public gender norms • Young women's disenfranchised position
	Does taking PrEP impact my sexuality in a negative way? *Ambivalences* concerning how PrEP may augment harmful sexual practices	• PrEP pushes the boundaries of sexuality and leads to chemsex (DK)	• Social and peer influence • Mental health of queer men
	Is PrEP safe in the long term? *Concerns* about the unknown long-term effects of PrEP	• Uncertainties about the long-term impact of PrEP on health (DK, Z) • Concerns about the long-term impacts of PrEP create caution around long-term use (DK)	• PrEP screening heightens attention to certain risks • Lack of information and knowledge

Table 2.3: Thematic network table of findings (continued)

Paradoxes	Everyday PrEP negotiations	Opposing ideas and 'ways of thinking' that give rise to contention, uncertainty, dilemmas, and ambiguity	Social context of ideas and 'ways of thinking' that mediate and amplify everyday PrEP negotiations
Liberating, yet constraining (PrEP is associated with a strong sense of sexual freedom and liberation, yet PrEP constrains in new ways)	Can I imagine a life without PrEP? *Held captive* by sexual freedom	• Addicted to the new lifestyle and status as a PrEP user (DK) • Strong sense of personal control over sexual health (DK)	• Collective fear of HIV and related stigma • The HIV 'at-risk' status and marginalisation of queer men
	What does PrEP require of me? *Considering* the constraints of PrEP treatment	• Keeping PrEP hidden is possible for some, but difficult for others (Z, DK) • Arduous pill-taking (Z, DK) • Too many demands and PrEP gets unattractive (Z)	• PrEP and sexuality stigma • Treatment regimen and the 'patient' persona required
	When should I stop taking PrEP? *Realising* the complexities of PrEP discontinuation	• Negotiating PrEP use with new partners (DK)	• Partner relations and communication • Norms around open relationships

Note: DK = Denmark; Z = Zimbabwe

THREE

Free, yet costly

The preceding chapters have set the stage for the empirical findings. In this chapter, I present one of the first paradoxes that PrEP users may encounter as they contemplate or seek out PrEP, namely that PrEP is *both* free *and* costly. This paradox captures opposing ideas and ways of thinking about PrEP as a medication that is available for free from national health services, yet that is also associated with significant costs, monetary or otherwise. The presence of such opposing and contradictory ideas necessitates different everyday PrEP negotiations. For queer men, public reminders of the fact that somebody foots the bill for PrEP triggered reflection on their privileged access to 'free' PrEP. Ambiguity arising from a lack of clarity around their deservedness prompted a need to justify and explain – to themselves and others – why PrEP should be free. For some young women in Zimbabwe, free PrEP access was associated with anticipated or actual out-of-pocket expenses. Due to their disenfranchised position, young women faced the dilemma of having to balance the value of PrEP, including the costs associated with PrEP access, with their perceived risk and needs. While out-of-pocket expenses were not considered an issue for our queer participants, the time spent accessing PrEP catalysed critical and contentious thinking about how PrEP services are organised.

This will be further discussed under the following headings:

- Why do I have free access? Making sense of privileged access to costly PrEP
- Is it really free? Balancing out-of-pocket expenses with HIV vulnerabilities
- Is free PrEP worth it? Thinking critically about PrEP service delivery

As explained earlier, the question in each heading introduces a contention, uncertainty, dilemma, or ambiguity. The question is followed by the type of everyday PrEP negotiation work that arises from this dialectic.

Why do I have free access? Making sense of privileged access to costly PrEP

In both contexts, study participants expressed awareness of and gratitude for the fact that PrEP was available for free through national health services. None of our participants took for granted that PrEP is freely available. They were acutely aware that somebody was footing the bill for PrEP, and many reflected on the reasons and circumstances leading to them having free PrEP. Erisy, a 24-year-old woman from Zimbabwe, for instance, reflected on the implications of health services not making PrEP available for free, alluding to the social inequalities that would arise from user payments:

> Imagine a scenario whereby PrEP was being sold to those who had a lot of money. This would inevitably mean that not everyone was going to afford it, and the poor would have continued getting infected with HIV. Keeping PrEP free allows us to protect ourselves from HIV, regardless of our background. (Erisy, age 24, eligible for PrEP)

Figure 3.1: More than a glass of water

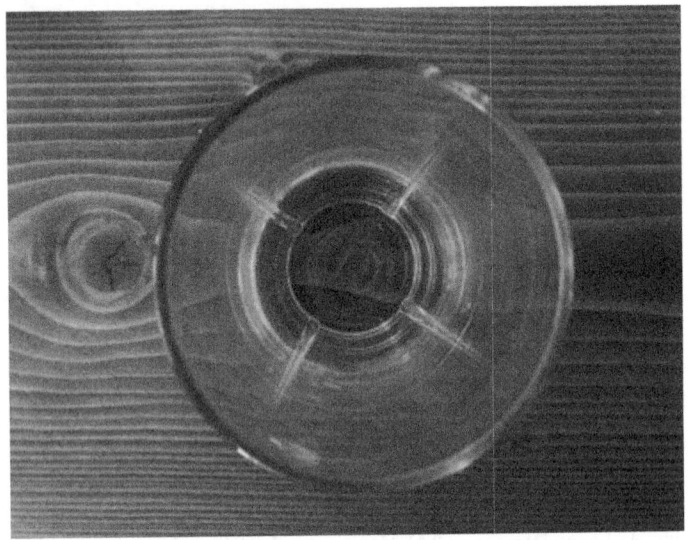

When queer men in Denmark expressed their appreciation of PrEP being free through national health services, they often spoke about it as a privilege. However, the notion and idea of PrEP being free and a privilege took different forms. José, a South American immigrant living in Copenhagen, describes how he is reminded, on a daily basis, of the privilege of living in a country where PrEP is freely available:

> This picture is of a glass of water (see Figure 3.1). It represents my daily routine of taking PrEP, which I consider to be a real privilege. I come from a country in South America that has limited resources, even to treat people living with HIV. It is difficult to get preventive pills like PrEP since it is not seen as a priority by the health authorities. I'm aware that there are other countries in Europe where PrEP is still not approved for common use. That's why I feel really privileged. I don't take the benefit of having free access to PrEP for granted. I admire

the Danish government for their decision to make this medicine available for all the members of the LGBTQI community. (José, age 33, PrEP user)

José is acutely aware that PrEP is a costly drug, and for that reason it is inaccessible to many of his peers in other countries. While transnational and global health inequalities in access cemented his ideas about privilege, for many of the queer men in our study, ideas of privilege were rooted in encounters with news reports detailing controversies around making PrEP freely available to individuals with an elevated chance of contracting HIV. Health economists and politicians have in the Danish media talked about the costs of PrEP and called for user payments, arguing that gay men should take responsibility for their own sex lives, and referred to condom use as a cheaper alternative. Such representations circulate in the public sphere and within the queer community, reminding queer men of the contested nature of their privileged access to free PrEP. Awareness of this contention forces queer men interested in or already taking PrEP to consider and justify their PrEP use against a backdrop of controversy, necessitating everyday PrEP negotiations. Sigurd, who is 35 and on PrEP, is one of the many queer men who expressed an awareness of the contested nature of PrEP being free. He was spending a lot of time and energy thinking about this, not least to come to an understanding and resolution through which this made sense to him. This included reflections on how the rigid controls and screening processes of PrEP eligibility in Denmark are in place because the drugs are expensive and there is a need to restrict PrEP access to a limited group of individuals vulnerable to HIV. It also included having to justify the legitimacy of his and other queer men's PrEP use. Sigurd projected exhaustion from having to deal with what he called 'societal stigma' around PrEP 'costing a lot of money' and the question 'why can't the gays not just use a condom?' Although he claimed that nobody in his immediate social network subscribed to these ideas, he did mention that he had had to justify and explain his PrEP use to peers. Sigurd appeared tired of having to explain why distributing PrEP for free is a good idea. However, he admitted he had done a lot of thinking around PrEP and its controversies, and despite finding it tiring, he felt a sense of responsibility to educate others about PrEP and its benefits.

Awareness of the contested nature of PrEP being free not only contributed to a sense of privilege. Queer men, like Sigurd, articulated ambiguity related to their deservedness of a costly drug like PrEP, instigating a need to understand, explain, and justify why free PrEP is a sound public health strategy, and why *they* are worth the expense. While the queer men participating in our study appeared able to do so, this form of everyday PrEP negotiation was rather exhausting for some. They recognised that not everyone eligible for PrEP may necessarily overcome internal contradictions, or reach the conclusion that they deserve free PrEP, meaning that some individuals warrant support and advocacy to deal with this ambivalence. This brings me to the next theme.

A few queer men also positioned PrEP in the broader historical context of fights for queer rights and access to services. They recognised that they were part of a larger community, and that other people had fought for their rights to be queer and proud, and to have access to sexual health services. Jens, who is 40 years old and eligible for and interested in PrEP, explains: 'I am part of a larger community which has a history of fighting for our rights, including access to PrEP. Indirectly I feel I have an obligation to continue this fight.' Jens does not take for granted that PrEP is available to him for free. He recognises the cost of past activist work and feels a sense of obligation to do his part in safeguarding the (fragile) rights of his community. This sense of obligation was central to the everyday PrEP negotiations of several of our queer participants. Aside from helping them give meaning to 'free' PrEP, it also meant that they, after enrolling onto PrEP, took an activist stance by disclosing their PrEP use, starting conversations about their sexuality and PrEP, and breaking down taboos.

Is it really free? Balancing out-of-pocket expenses with HIV vulnerabilities

For our young female participants in Zimbabwe, many of whom live in poverty, access was associated with out-of-pocket expenses, shaping their perspectives about the costs of accessing 'free' PrEP. Two costs were frequently mentioned. First, there was a common understanding that PrEP was not accessible from local clinics and that they had to travel further afield. It was not uncommon to hear from the women that 'the distance is far and getting a bus fare can be challenging', as described by 22-year-old Precious. Monica, who participated in a focus group discussion, went on to detail how her husband would refuse to provide her with money for a bus fare:

> Going to the clinic requires a bus fare because the clinic is far from where I live. I do not have the money, and my husband will start making excuses that he doesn't have money for transport either. I will thus decide that it's better not go to the clinic. (Monica, age 18–24, PrEP interested)

For some young women like Monica, the out-of-pocket expenses related to accessing free PrEP were a reminder of their dependency on their male partners and ultimately their disenfranchised position. The role of gender orders and norms in shaping PrEP access and use among young women is a dominant and recurrent theme that I will return to in all subsequent chapters.

The second out-of-pocket expense mentioned by a few of the young women related to hospital or consultation fees, which, although often limited to US$1, were described as prohibitive for those with limited financial resources. The fee is charged upon entering the health facility for registration and referral to the relevant department. The notion that the US$1 consultation fee is prohibitive was a common theme in our interviews with healthcare providers, who strongly recommended the elimination of all out-of-pocket expenses associated with PrEP access (Skovdal et al., 2022b). These out-of-pocket expenses appeared to require some young women to weigh up conflicting priorities. Money spent on accessing 'free' PrEP, whether it related to transport or hospital administration fees, was money taken away from other, perhaps more pressing expenditures, such as feeding their children. Such considerations may be further complicated by perceptions of PrEP unavailability. A few young women said that there was no guarantee that PrEP would be available at the hospital, which may have made them err on the side of not spending out-of-pocket money to access it. Ideas about PrEP being unavailable, added to the cost of accessing PrEP by either having to travel further afield or return to the clinic at a later time, tap into a shared experience of local clinics being poorly stocked. As part of their everyday PrEP negotiations, young women had to pensively navigate the dilemma of having to weigh up their chances of contracting HIV and ideas of 'free' PrEP against the perception that PrEP is unobtainable due to a combination of out-of-pocket expenses, gender norms, and other competing life demands.

None of the queer men in Denmark who participated in our study spoke about out-of-pocket expenses as a hinderance to their access, partly reflecting their high income context and the fact that we were unable to recruit participants from more deprived sectors of Danish society.

Is free PrEP worth it? Thinking critically about PrEP service delivery

While participants in both contexts talked about time as an opportunity cost associated with accessing PrEP, time spent accessing 'free' PrEP shaped much of the data with queer men in Denmark. Many ascribed to the idea that PrEP services are severely restricted in terms of geographical accessibility and opening hours. As described in Chapter 2, PrEP services in Denmark are highly centralised and restricted to the nine hospitals in Denmark that have infectious disease departments, five of which are in Copenhagen or its vicinity. Most of the queer men we spoke to lived in Copenhagen and in theory did not have to travel far. Nonetheless, many still spoke about the inconvenience of having to go to hospital during working hours. Mike and Christian described this inconvenience, but they both recognised that they have jobs that offer flexibility and that make it possible for them to attend appointments in the middle of the day. They reflected on this privilege, and Mike noted that for people living further away, the opportunity costs associated with PrEP access may be too great:

> I think it's really inconvenient to go to Hvidovre Hospital. To get some medicine and get some tests done which … my doctor in principle can do, right? It's something that I find difficult in my everyday life. That I have to take half a day off almost, to get all the way out there […] I'm always thinking of someone who doesn't live in Copenhagen. If you live elsewhere, would you then have to take a full day off work? (Mike, age 32, PrEP user)

> To get to the infectious disease department, I have to cycle 11 kilometers each way and often spend one to two hours in the hospital, but only really talk to the nurse for two minutes. I do the tests for STDs myself and a nurse takes blood samples. I'm so privileged that I can move my work around and find time to go to the hospital. I feel like I'm spending a lot of time on something that could be a lot easier. The consultation could for example be done online, and the tests could definitely be done at a hospital closer to me or at my GP. (Christian, age 26, PrEP user)

While centralised PrEP services and restricted opening hours are an inconvenience for Mike and Christian, they acknowledge that these factors pose a significant barrier to PrEP uptake for others. Other participants discussed the difficulties of asking their manager for time off to attend a PrEP consultation and expressed concerns that they might have to explain to colleagues (if asked) where they are going. For queer men with a precarious attachment to the labour market, such factors were especially challenging.

What such accounts underline is that the PrEP pills do not just fall into the laps of queer men. Yes, PrEP is available for free from the hospital, but accessing the medication comes at an expense to their time, whether it is taking the time to travel or taking time off work to go to the hospital. Mike took a photo of his local pharmacy to express his dissatisfaction that PrEP pills cannot be collected at pharmacies (see Figure 6.3, Chapter 6). Another queer man aired the idea of introducing a small user-fee if it meant he could pick up his drugs at a local pharmacy. For him, the opportunity costs associated with the way 'free' PrEP is delivered in Denmark outweighed a potential actual cost of the pill. There are evidently competing interests at stake, giving rise to contention and critical thinking.

National health services have an interest in centralising PrEP services, whereas some queer men are keen to decentralise PrEP services, making PrEP more easily accessible. This contention is the source of many everyday PrEP negotiations. Our queer participants spent a lot of time thinking and talking about the rigidity of PrEP services in Denmark and how this contributes to significant opportunity costs. They appreciated the fact that PrEP is freely available, but also considered time as a valuable resource and a cost that has to be factored into accessing 'free' PrEP. This sparked critical thinking and encouraged them to discuss with each other how PrEP services could be delivered differently.

While many queer men expressed a strong desire for the decentralisation of PrEP services, many participants also reported negative experiences with testing for sexually transmitted infections or obtaining referrals for PrEP from their general practitioners, due to both stigma and a lack of knowledge about PrEP among general practitioners. This may seem contradictory, but it suggests that queer men are at different stages of their PrEP journey. As I further illustrate in Chapter 5, queer men who are new to PrEP – perhaps because they are young and in the process of coming to terms with their sexuality – need safe and queer-friendly health services, which are most likely achieved by more centralised and specialised services. In contrast, queer men who are seasoned PrEP users and have grown confident and comfortable with their sexuality through strong social support may be better equipped to handle potential stigma or ignorance from decentralised PrEP services and therefore prefer this over centralised services. Either way, this highlights the need for more differentiated PrEP services that adapt delivery to better meet the dynamic and changing realities of individuals (WHO, 2022).

Concerns about time use and restricted opening hours were also mentioned by some of the young women in Zimbabwe. A few argued that adolescent and school-going girls would struggle to access PrEP within the existing clinic opening hours (typically from 8 am to 4 pm), as it would necessitate them skipping school. Time was a big issue for the young women. They expressed real concerns about the limited clinic opening hours, the amount of time it takes time to get to the clinic, and the waiting time once there. It was repeatedly stated that this conflicted with the time they needed to spend on income-generating activities or other household duties, as described by Judith, a young woman interested in PrEP: 'I am still struggling to find the time to go there [the PrEP clinic] because I have a lot of household duties to do, so for me to find time to visit the clinic is proving difficult.'

Judith – as part of her everyday PrEP negotiations – has actively thought about and analysed the pros and cons of investing the time to go and access 'free' PrEP. She has concluded that, for now, given the time it will take to access PrEP, it is not a feasible HIV prevention method for her. By

FOUR

Eligible, yet ineligible

The second paradox covered in this book relates to contradictory ideas about PrEP eligibility. Many of our study participants in both case studies described having to navigate ideas about their being *both* eligible *and* ineligible for PrEP depending on who gets to define, or have a voice and a decision in, their PrEP use. Many of our study participants recognised their eligibility for PrEP because of their affiliation to a PrEP target group and their chance of contracting HIV. Yet – again, in both our case studies – many people in society in general and also among their immediate family and friends either considered them ineligible or sought to maintain their ineligibility by reproducing stigmatising representations of who a PrEP user is. This was especially the case for young women in Zimbabwe who encountered ideas and points of view that made them question or renounce their PrEP eligibility. Many parents and male partners objected to these young women's PrEP use, demonstrating the presence of cultural eligibility criteria. For queer men in Denmark, tensions around (in)eligibility focused on a mismatch between their ideas of eligibility and those detailed in policy frameworks and applied by PrEP service providers. Many of our queer male participants did not meet the official criteria for PrEP eligibility and spoke about the need to wilfully lie to PrEP service providers in order to access PrEP. Regardless of context, opposing and diverging understandings of PrEP (in)eligibility were omnipresent and gave rise to numerous everyday PrEP negotiations in the form of dealing with stigma, with both the queer men and the young women having to consider their responses to, and the consequences of, the efforts they had to make to negotiate their own eligibility. These will be discussed under the following headings:

- Are 'good girls' on PrEP? Considering cultural eligibility criteria
- How will others view my eligibility? Fearing stigmatising associations with PrEP use
- Should I lie or appeal for flexibility? Navigating 'the system' and negotiating eligibility

Are 'good girls' on PrEP? Considering cultural eligibility criteria

As already mentioned, most of the young women participating in our Zimbabwe study considered themselves eligible for PrEP. The married young women in particular talked about their chances of contracting HIV from their husbands, whom many strongly suspected – or even expected – to be unfaithful. The women spoke positively about PrEP and recognised its unique potential to protect them against HIV, particularly when condom use is difficult to negotiate. While sexually active adolescent girls and young women are eligible for PrEP from health services in Zimbabwe, it is evident from our young female participants that these are not the only criteria they need to navigate. PrEP's signalling of sexuality required young women who live with a partner or husband, or at home with parents, to consider cultural eligibility criteria. Premarital and extramarital sex is frowned upon in this cultural context and challenges gender norms and ideas about what it means to be a 'good girl'. Illustrating the impact of collective understandings of what it means to be a 'good girl', many young women, such as 20-year-old Rosey, spoke about their parents' disapproval of them having sex if unmarried: 'I am not yet married so in their eyes I am not supposed to be having sex at this point.' Ellena expanded on this in a description of a photograph (see Figure 4.1):

> This is a picture of two older people. A man and a woman. And I took it to represent a mother and a father with children who are adolescents or young adults. The way our society is set up, parents will never acknowledge that their children are having sex especially if they are not yet married. This then implies that they are not expected to be using any HIV prevention methods. This counts as a discouraging factor for the children because they then fear judgement from their parents and end up not protecting themselves from HIV by taking up PrEP. (Ellena, age 21, eligible for PrEP)

Strong collective understandings of the need for unmarried girls to refrain from having sex meant that many of our young female participants articulated a shared belief that parents do not consider unmarried young women eligible for PrEP.

Figure 4.1: Fear of judgement from parents

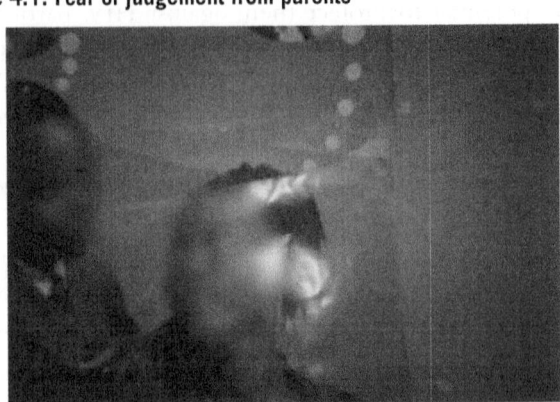

Adding to this disapproval, Memory noted in a focus group discussion that 'parents also won't accept PrEP because this promotes promiscuity', highlighting a fear that PrEP may further legitimise and reproduce promiscuous behaviours. In another focus group discussion, Janice, who is eligible for PrEP and within the 18–24-year age range, shared: 'Even grandmothers you will be staying with will deny you access to PrEP because they will be saying that their child is clean and so, accessing PrEP will result in promiscuity which is not allowed by our grandmothers.'

The idea that parents do not want their girl-children to engage with PrEP was prominent and not wholly unfounded. Elsewhere we report on parents' attitudes towards PrEP and find a mix of positive and negative attitudes towards PrEP (Skovdal et al., 2023). This suggests that parents may be more accepting of PrEP than is commonly believed among our young female participants. However, parents who reported having accepting attitudes towards PrEP still struggled to reconcile this with the traditional gender norms of what it means to be a 'good girl' (Skovdal et al., 2023), underlining the cultural dismissal of PrEP for 'good girls'. A few young women went on to try and explain where these 'good girl' notions come from, often referring to either culture or religion. Ellena, in a description of a photograph she took of a church poster (see Figure 4.2), details her belief that religious leaders play a central role in promoting the public gender norms that govern young women's sexuality:

> The second picture I took was of a church poster with a pastor and his wife. These are religious leaders who act as our moral compasses in our communities. Church leaders set standards for behaviour that is acceptable and for behaviour which is not acceptable. They police sexual behaviour and frown upon what they define as being against the word of God. So when looking at barriers to the uptake of PrEP, church leaders play a key role.

They preach abstinence as the only way expected from unmarried people. (Ellena, age 21, eligible for PrEP)

Married young women expected similar dismissals of their PrEP eligibility from their husbands. While a few young women could, from personal experience, describe having support from their husbands, many others noted that their husbands were likely to disapprove of their PrEP use. Some women explained that their PrEP use would be interpreted by their husbands or male partners as either a signal of the women's infidelity or as distrust of their partner. As a result, this led to the common understanding, as articulated by Tanya, that young women will 'fail to be on PrEP because their husbands will not approve of it'.

PrEP has been hailed as a female-controlled HIV prevention method, but our data highlight that before young women get to the point of accessing PrEP, they have to navigate disapproving attitudes rooted in a symbolic context of cultural expectations and representations of what it means to be a 'good girl'. While most young women in our study were able to personally resist this representation and saw 'good girls' as those who were able

Figure 4.2: A church poster

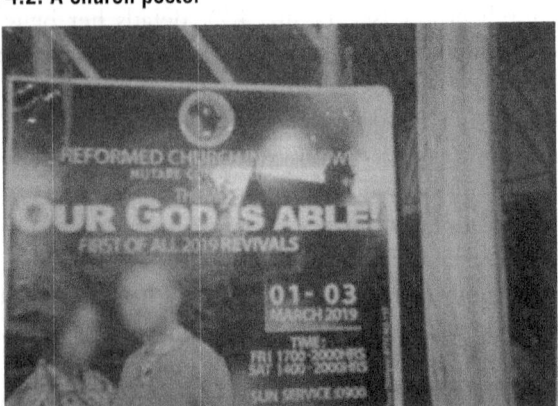

to protect themselves and others from HIV, collective meanings, and interpretations of how parents and partners might negatively react to their PrEP use, highlight the need for everyday PrEP negotiations. Young women must consider and work out parent or partner attitudes towards PrEP, their anticipated reactions, as well as the consequences of being discovered to be a PrEP user.

In the next section I discuss how 'good girl' notions are often enforced through PrEP-related stigma, which young women must also navigate and negotiate in everyday life.

How will others view my eligibility? Fearing stigmatising associations with PrEP use

Many young women also feared PrEP-related stereotypes, such as PrEP's association with women with so-called loose morals or prostitute traits. PrEP was often referred to as being an HIV prevention method for sex workers. This understanding is not entirely baseless and reflects the fact that more than half of the people who were offered oral PrEP in Zimbabwe following its introduction in 2016 were female sex workers (Ministry of Health and Child Care, 2018). However, sex work is highly stigmatised. One female PrEP user in Zimbabwe captures how she is confronted with stigmatising ideas about PrEP because of it being, among other things, associated with sex work. She explains how this connection challenges her engagement with PrEP services:

> Being a young woman on PrEP in our community is difficult because people are conservative and do not know that PrEP helps. I face challenges accessing PrEP. People think that I am on antiretroviral therapy, yet I am not. Many people are saying I am a sex worker, yet I am not. This becomes a challenge when I am going to collect PrEP at the hospital. As a young woman it is difficult to be on PrEP because in the community, they are not accepting me properly. (Stephanie, age 23, PrEP user)

For Stephanie, PrEP's association with sex work challenges her engagement with the drug. However, as she also notes, stigmatising attitudes about who a PrEP user is, including PrEP's association with sex work, make it generally very difficult for women in her community to access PrEP. As there is a requirement for female sexuality to be considered 'virtuous' in this cultural setting, it is only a short step from the cultural 'anxiety' and 'panic' associated with HIV prevention methods that allow girls to be sexual (that is, in 'virtuous' contexts such as marriage, or indeed before marriage), to representing PrEP use as irresponsible and immoral. Stephanie also alludes to PrEP's association with HIV treatment. Being a daily pill, collected from the same sexual infection departments that administer antiretroviral therapy for treatment of HIV, led to representations of PrEP as a cover-up for treatment. In other words, if you are a young woman on PrEP, people in the community may assume that you live with HIV and are on treatment for the virus. While Stephanie had managed to ignore or deal with social representations of PrEP as being either for sex workers or a cover for HIV treatment, it was an issue she had had to confront and continued to encounter.

Most of the young women in our study were not on PrEP, but were eligible and considering it. They too had thought about the anticipated implications of stigmatising attitudes affecting their engagement. Rachel, who is 25 years old and eligible for PrEP, explains: 'People are scared of taking PrEP because the tablets look like the ones that are taken by HIV positive people, so one may be scared of what people will say about the person taking tablets that are similar to that.'

Stephanie's interview captured a series of everyday PrEP negotiations, spanning mental activities and partner interactions. Through an analysis and interpretation of how HIV-related stigma has evolved in her community, Stephanie believes that the stigmatisation of PrEP users will soon come to an end: 'I just told myself that people talked about those [people] on antiretroviral therapy [ART], and it [the feeling of stigmatisation] stopped.' Stephanie also engages in an 'othering' of stigmatisers, demonstrating a cognitive bias against those whom she perceives as different or less knowledgeable than her: 'People say things without proper understanding.' Finally, she has involved her husband in her decision-making, resulting in him knowing about and approving her PrEP use: 'My husband is aware that I am taking PrEP.' Through everyday PrEP negotiations, Stephanie has actively confronted stigmatising attitudes triggered by PrEP user representations. This confronting of stigmatising attitudes was also demonstrated by Angela, a 23-year-old PrEP user, who explained: 'There are others who believe that PrEP is a form of ART [antiretroviral therapy] and that people who take it are brainwashed into believing it is for HIV positive people. But because we know what PrEP does, we try to correct their perception about it.'

Stigma linked to PrEP is rife. While some young women like Stephanie and Angela manage to navigate stigmatising attitudes and do their best to combat PrEP-related stigma, it is a barrier to PrEP interest, access, and uptake for many others. PrEP-related stigma requires young women who are interested in PrEP to carefully consider and think through the potential consequences of accessing PrEP from their local clinic. Precious, Megan, and Hope, three young women who consider themselves eligible for PrEP, detail their understandings of how local clinics and the way PrEP is administered constrain their ability to take it up. Precious describes difficulties in taking PrEP discreetly, highlighting the likelihood that someone will recognise her and that word will spread that she is on PrEP:

> When you get to where the pill is accessed, you may see a relative or someone from the community. If they see me leaving the place with a pill box where it's written PrEP, they will go back to the community and tell them that I am taking PrEP. (Precious, age 22, eligible for PrEP)

> Girls would be shy to go and look for HIV prevention methods at the hospital because everyone will know that she is having sex, and she will be labeled a loose woman. (Megan, age 20, eligible for PrEP)

Along related lines, others represented PrEP service providers as being indiscreet and likely to inform parents that their girl-child is seeking out PrEP. When women toyed with the idea of taking PrEP discreetly, the risks associated with parents or partners discovering their PrEP use were often stated as superseding the benefits of PrEP. This and the social risks of PrEP use are discussed in detail in Chapter 7.

Another issue raised by the women was the attitude of some healthcare providers. Healthcare providers were on occasion represented as being part and parcel of the community, thus holding the same conservative and judgemental views as their parents, and therefore actively discouraging adolescent girls from taking up PrEP:

> Young girls fear going to the nearest clinics because of their age, and service providers asking her why she is coming to the clinic to get HIV prevention methods like PrEP and condoms at such a young age. She will end up having unprotected sex and not using any other HIV prevention methods because she will be fearing to go to the nearest clinic where the service providers are judgemental. (Hope, age 24, eligible for PrEP)

The focus of this chapter thus far has been on young women in Zimbabwe. They form part of a collectivist culture, and their everyday PrEP negotiations are characterised by having to consider the interests, wishes, and expectations of the people around them. So, while the young women in our study recognise their eligibility for PrEP – meeting the criteria set out by health services in Zimbabwe – they are compelled to also consider another set of more culturally embedded criteria that dictate that only girls with 'loose morals' or 'prostitute traits' are eligible. PrEP is supposedly redundant for 'good girls', rendering them ineligible for it. Practically, this means that people around them, and even PrEP service providers who side with cultural criteria for eligibility, are perceived to not consider them eligible, thus challenging their access to and engagement with PrEP. It also means that some young women struggle to ascertain their eligibility. On the one hand, they consider themselves to be 'good girls', albeit perhaps using different standards to those of their parents, partners, and the broader community; on the other hand, they recognise their chances of contracting HIV. Young women may therefore find themselves battling ideas about their (in)eligibility – having to negotiate their own eligibility, and navigate (and reject) their community's cultural desires and expectations of them as being ineligible.

Eligibility also has to be negotiated by queer men in Denmark. To limit the number of people on PrEP, driven by there being a cap on PrEP financing within the Danish national health services, only individuals who are demonstrably vulnerable to HIV are eligible for PrEP. However, queer men who fail to meet the strict criteria detailed in policy frameworks may still consider themselves eligible, albeit from a self- and community-defined HIV vulnerability perspective. As I will show in the next section, these diverging understandings of (in)eligibility trigger everyday PrEP negotiations geared to help queer men navigate, or even manipulate, 'the system' to access PrEP.

Should I lie or appeal for flexibility? Navigating 'the system' and negotiating eligibility

PrEP services in both Denmark and Zimbabwe operate within a policy framework with guidelines detailing how PrEP should be delivered and who qualifies for it. Given resource constraints, such guidelines have been devised to focus on those most vulnerable to HIV, optimising impact and value for money.

At the time of our Zimbabwe study, PrEP had only recently been rolled out for adolescent girls and young women. As such, some of the young women participating in our study, despite knowing they are part of the target group, questioned their own eligibility, thinking that the limited stock of drugs should be preserved for young women more vulnerable to HIV than them. As noted by Zendaya in a focus group discussion, this perception also contributed to the idea that young women would be questioned about their sexuality when seeking PrEP, which would make them feel intimidated and embarrassed:

> According to my own understanding on PrEP, it is not yet readily available to all clinics in this community and even if it is accessed from the clinics, special preference is given to those who are at a higher risk of HIV. So, if it is a young person who has gone to the clinic to access PrEP, they may feel intimidated being asked a lot of questions. Some may even feel embarrassed with the questions that the nurses will be asking, and then decide that it's not worth the effort. (Zendaya, in the age group 18–24, eligible for PrEP)

Zendaya further notes that the anticipation of having to justify and explain one's eligibility for PrEP may be off-putting for some young women, who may then simply decide not to seek out PrEP. She also points to a discomfort in having to explain and justify this eligibility. She captures some of the thinking and considerations that go into the decision of young women to seek out PrEP. Such everyday PrEP negotiations are undoubtedly also applicable to some queer men in Denmark who are considering PrEP but are unsure if they meet the official criteria and have little interest in talking about their sex life. However, for our queer participants, most of whom are already on PrEP, the focus was on how they navigated 'the system' and negotiated their eligibility, which may or may not be aligned with official guidelines.

Queer men in Denmark spoke at length about their concerns about not meeting official criteria for PrEP eligibility. However, rather than necessarily seeing rigid criteria as something that prevents them from accessing PrEP, several queer men directed their negotiation efforts into making sense of, and critiquing, what they considered a broken system for determining eligibility. They also sought to find ways to navigate the system and negotiated a new understanding of eligibility – one that differs from the official policy framework.

The reason for all this everyday PrEP negotiation work comes down to competing interests and opposing ideas about the aim of PrEP. From the perspective of the Danish national health service, PrEP is a public health measure aimed solely at preventing HIV transmission among individuals vulnerable to the virus. In the context of a national health service, this needs to be achieved in the most cost-effective way. It is accomplished by applying rigid eligibility criteria that stipulate that queer men must have had unprotected anal intercourse with at least two male partners within the last 12 weeks, or acquired syphilis, chlamydia, or gonorrhoea within the last 24 weeks. For the PrEP service providers I have spoken to, the motivation to apply eligibility criteria comes down to the principle of 'do no harm', meaning they do not wish to prescribe PrEP medication to someone who is not vulnerable to HIV. However – as I demonstrate in forthcoming chapters – for many queer men, PrEP is much more than a method for reducing HIV incidence within a population group. PrEP provides comfort and safety; it liberates and makes having sex fun again; it removes the black cloud of fear that has tainted queer sexuality for decades; it provides a community and social identity. For some, PrEP removes the shame of queer sex, and for others it supports a long-standing promise to their parents not to contract HIV. Queer men's recognition of what PrEP offers above and beyond reducing HIV incidence within their community is attractive. However, queer men who are unable to demonstrate their vulnerabilities based on past behaviour are ineligible. So are queer men who have the intention of taking more risk. The limited scope of the official criteria with regards to past and high-risk behaviour was considered nonsensical by many of our queer participants. They referred to it as a chicken-and-egg situation and expressed frustration that 'the system' requires them to take risks before qualifying for PrEP. Both Jens and Sigurd raise what they consider the absurdity of not being able to pre-empt risk, and of future intentions or probabilities not being considered:

> I was at the clinic six months ago, and the PrEP provider told me that I was not slutty enough to be given PrEP. For a long time, I have found it amusing that you need to drive 140km/h without a seatbelt to be eligible for PrEP, and where it may be too late. (Jens, age 40, awaiting PrEP)

> If you knew that there was a high probability that you are going to do it, it would be very nice to be able to take care of yourself beforehand. (Sigurd, age 35, PrEP user)

Queer men who in the past have done everything in their power to limit their risk of HIV but aspire to having more adventurous and fulfilling sex lives, either by increasing their number of sexual partners or by looking to have condomless anal sex, do not meet the official eligibility criteria. They know that continuing 'on the high road' does not grant them PrEP. Jens, who six months prior to his interview for this study was denied access to PrEP, reportedly changed his sexual behaviour to meet the eligibility criteria: 'I went back three weeks ago. My sex life has changed […] I answered some of the questions differently, which made her conclude that I was totally eligible. I am now waiting for a call, confirming my referral.' Given the diversity of his more recent sexual practices, Jens goes on to claim that he was not put in a position of having to lie. However, if he had to lie to access PrEP, he now knows what to say and would not hesitate to embellish his past sexuality:

> I am not going to lie to get PrEP, because I have no need to. But if I find myself in a situation where I have to, in order to access PrEP, I will tell them that I have fucked four guys in the past six months without condom. I know that is what I have to say to get PrEP. (Jens, age 40, awaiting PrEP)

'Knowing what to say' to access PrEP may sound like an easy way to 'work the system'. But for many of our queer participants, having to lie was not something they did lightly or felt comfortable sharing. Both Christian and Toke, who were otherwise articulate throughout their interviews, stumbled over their words and thoughts in their struggle to say that they had lied about their sexuality to access PrEP:

> Well, when I came for an interview at … the hospital, uh. Then we talked about it and like um … And then, to be sure that I would get it, I just said … what they wanted to hear. Uh, that I had uhh, unprotected sex with a lot of people. And then I got it … like um … yes. […] there I think maybe I was a little … yes, nervous that I like … wouldn't get it if I like … had … had talked a little more honestly about my sex life, or something like that, or … Well, I didn't quite know how much it would take to … to get it. (Christian, age 26, PrEP user)

> I, like, could read that there were some criteria. So, in practical terms, it's about having a … a … I mean, a sexual behaviour with frequent unprotected sex. And … at the time, I didn't actually … I mean, I did not actually meet the criteria. So … I lied, you might say. I knew what I had to say, and then I got the medicine. You could say that my sexual behaviour has changed

since. I have become more active, and now I meet the
criteria [laughter]. (Toke, age 27, PrEP user)

Christian and Toke both knew they did not strictly meet the criteria for PrEP, and entered the PrEP initiation process knowing they had to embellish the truth about their past sexual practices in order to access PrEP. Some participants spoke about how they had received advice from PrEP-using peers to just 'say what they want to hear', and others had heard that some PrEP providers were more lenient in their interpretation of the guidelines. Specific names of nurses and doctors known to also consider future vulnerabilities to HIV in their assessment circulated within some of the queer men's peer networks. As such, young men like Christian, who are looking to start taking PrEP, either need to read the situation and pick up on subtle cues in order to say 'what it will take to get it', or actively seek out named PrEP service providers who are known for their leniency.

These everyday PrEP negotiations are justified, normalised, and enabled through users' interactions with peers and in social networks, where they talk about the so-called absurdity of having to take risks before being able to access PrEP. Although they lie with unease and feel uncomfortable talking about it in a recorded interview, their intentions of reaping the benefits of PrEP – which for some, like Toke, include more sexual risk-taking in the future – make them approach eligibility very differently from the policy frameworks that PrEP service providers enact. Nonetheless, these diverging understandings – including what comes first, the chicken (demonstrated vulnerabilities to HIV) or the egg (risk intention) – shape paradoxical ideas about (in)eligibility, which queer men have to carefully navigate, not least as they mentally prepare themselves for their PrEP prescribing consultation and the need to wilfully lie and navigate their way to eligibility. While our queer participants succeeded in this endeavour, others may not have the support network or stamina to enter an appointment with healthcare staff knowing that they must lie to access PrEP, thus creating inequalities in access.

Opposing ideas about PrEP (in)eligibility were also expressed by some of the young women in Zimbabwe. Here, too, contention was a result of rigid understandings of who qualifies for PrEP. However, unlike the experiences of queer men having to deceive and work 'the system', young women in Zimbabwe alluded to eligibility criteria being more amenable to renegotiation. One example is from Angela, who described how she managed to renegotiate the terms around her PrEP use by convincing healthcare staff that her husband should also be deemed eligible and have access to PrEP:

> When I approached PrEP services, I asked them if my husband could also take the pills because that would be the only way I could take the pills. They were adamant that only women are taking the pills, but I explained my situation, that we are open to each other, and I would not want to hide this from him. I would rather take the tablets with my husband with no secrets. After a while they agreed that my husband can take the pills. I then went home and told my husband who was okay with this, and we went back, got tested, counselled, and initiated onto PrEP. (Angela, age 23, PrEP user)

Unlike many young women in Manicaland, Zimbabwe, Angela can talk openly about PrEP with her partner, which she considers a prerequisite for her eligibility. Angela's account ties back to some of the issues discussed earlier in the chapter, underlining PrEP use in Zimbabwe as a profoundly gendered practice (see Chapter 2 for the background of gender orders in Zimbabwe) that gives rise to many considerations and negotiations.

Conclusion

This chapter has shown that there are different and diverging ideas about what constitutes (in)eligibility for PrEP. Young

FIVE

Responsible, yet irresponsible

This chapter discusses the third paradox of the book, namely the notion that PrEP users are *both* responsible *and* irresponsible with regards to their sexual health. This paradox relates primarily to queer men in Denmark, who, on the one hand, recognise how PrEP supports them in their efforts to take responsibility for preventing HIV, yet, on the other hand, brings them to encounter ideas that associate PrEP with irresponsible sexual behaviour. The idea of being responsible appears to be rooted in an understanding of the difficulties in using condoms consistently, vulnerability to HIV, and the value of halting the spread of HIV. Meanwhile, associations between PrEP and irresponsible sexual behaviour stem from social representations of PrEP as being linked to risk compensation in the form of increased promiscuity and condomless anal sex, which in turn, despite evidence to the contrary (Murchu et al., 2022), are believed to contribute to a rise in other sexually transmitted infections. These opposing ideas are encountered in social interactions and inevitably draw on diverging socio-cultural views on queer sex and morality. For many of our participants, such opposing ideas were amplified and became particularly visible when hookups (that is, casual sexual encounters) and condom use were negotiated on mobile dating apps. What in general, and what particular ideas about (ir)responsible sexual behaviour, came to affect our participants was highly dependent on their social networks. It was through social networks that certain ideas and ways of thinking were challenged and reconstructed, and new and different ways of talking about PrEP were encountered. Noticeably, while young women in Zimbabwe felt ashamed to access PrEP, as discussed in the previous chapter, none of them talked about PrEP being associated with irresponsibility regarding sexual health. Although I will make a few references to young women in Zimbabwe, this chapter primarily draws on the accounts and experiences of queer men in Denmark.

The dialectics arising from PrEP's association with both responsible and irresponsible sexual health behaviour necessitate numerous everyday PrEP negotiations. I capture and explore these through the following three headings:

- Am I taking responsibility for my sexual health? Negotiating 'PrEP responsibility' in a relational context
- Why do I feel irresponsible when taking responsibility? Shame associated with PrEP
- Am *I* irresponsible? 'Othering' non-PrEP users

Am I taking responsibility for my sexual health? Negotiating 'PrEP responsibility' in a relational context

All participants across the two study settings subscribed to the idea that PrEP represents taking responsibility for one's own sexual health and that of others. However, ideas about PrEP also being linked to *irresponsible* sexual behaviour were omnipresent among our queer male participants. Charles, who is interested in PrEP, talked about the social representation of PrEP being linked to promiscuity:

> Taking PrEP is seen a little bit like a licence to be – if not promiscuous – to be sexually active [little laugh].

> There are some in the gay community, who because of internalised homophobia, consider people on PrEP as 'too gay'. Too ready to have gay sex. Promiscuous. (Charles, age 65, eligible for PrEP)

What Charles is also alluding to is divisions within the queer community, and how PrEP spurs new ideas of (ir)responsibility and queerness. These ideas appear to be encountered and amplified by certain relational practices, such as negotiating condom use and using dating apps for hookups, which will be the focus on this section.

I would like to begin with our participants' relationship to condoms. There was a broad and shared understanding that using condoms consistently is impossible, and it is in the context of this representation that taking PrEP becomes a responsible thing to do. The queer men in Denmark often referred to the belief that using condoms in 'the heat of the moment' is challenging. Jens, a 40-year-old man who was not on PrEP at the time of the study but awaiting a referral, explains that he only uses condoms half the time: '*I think it's impractical. I think it's a turn-off in that act.*' Young women in Zimbabwe also occasionally referred to the challenge of using condoms in the 'heat of the moment' but did so in relation to how much access there is to condoms. Maidei, in her account of the role of PrEP in HIV prevention, took a photograph of a condom (see Figure 5.1) and described the common idea that young people do not have access to condoms as and when they need them, and that young women do not always have the power to negotiate condom use with men:

> This is a picture of a pack of condoms. Condoms are the traditional and old way of protecting against HIV that almost everyone in our communities know about, even the young children – they grow up knowing that there is something called condoms. The importance of PrEP comes out for me when looking at this condom

because I feel that one of the reasons young people end up getting HIV is the fact that they sometimes do not have access to condoms at the very moment they want to have sexual intercourse. I can imagine a situation whereby two young people meet up and they are now in the heat of the moment wanting sex, but they have no condoms with them. If one is already on PrEP it means they are protected, even if they have sex without condoms, they will maintain their negative status. The other thing with this condom is that it is worn by men and they have the power to protect. If a man decides he does not want to use condoms it means the female counterpart is at risk of having HIV. If she is already on PrEP she would have protected herself from getting HIV. (Maidei, age 26, eligible for PrEP)

Many young women also referred to the point that married women face challenges in negotiating condom use with husbands. This is exemplified by Precious, who says that PrEP allows you to 'safeguard your health and life knowing that your husband is unfaithful'. It is against this background of ideas

Figure 5.1: Condom

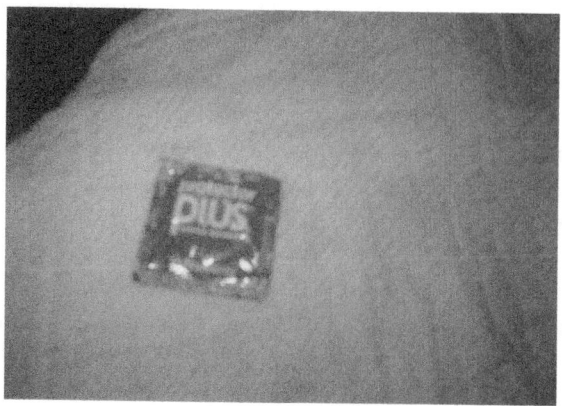

and beliefs about the practical limits of condoms that PrEP becomes synonymous with taking responsibility for one's own health and life.

Some queer male PrEP users who engaged in condomless anal sex expressed ambivalence in relation to how PrEP use affected their sexual behaviour. Poul, a 46-year-old PrEP user, describes how PrEP has allowed him to have casual sex responsibly because he does not have to worry about HIV. At the same time, he is acutely aware that having casual and condomless anal sex with different men increases his chances of contracting and spreading sexually transmitted infections, which he refers to as 'careless' behaviour:

> It [PrEP] allows me to have casual sex with random men in random places. Without having to think about HIV. But what about all the other sexually transmitted infections I can acquire? Why take PrEP at all if I have to put on a condom anyway to avoid everything else? After all, I don't put on both rainwear and an umbrella when it rains. PrEP has made me careless in some ways. I do just like everyone else – forget that there is also something other than HIV in circulation. (Poul, age 46, PrEP user)

Paul highlights an inherent paradox of the PrEP pill, namely that it protects (against HIV), yet it does not (against other sexually transmitted infections). For Poul, 'careless' or 'irresponsible' condomless anal sex is built into using PrEP. Combining PrEP and condom use is, to him, illogical. Why be on PrEP if you are using condoms anyway? While the impracticality of consistent condom use, as discussed earlier, justifies PrEP use, Poul's deliberations over how PrEP affects his sexual behaviour and condom use illustrate how such opposing ideas affect self-understandings (for example, being 'careless'), thoughts, and actions. Many queer male PrEP users in Denmark encountered these ideas on Grindr, a dating app, which cemented different types of (ir)responsibility. For Klaus, a 42-year-old queer man in an open polyamorous relationship, PrEP simply represents taking responsibility for sexual health: one's own and others'. He says, 'If I can see on the app that he is on PrEP, I feel safer.' He goes on to argue that if he is contacted by someone on Grindr who is not on PrEP, he will approach a possible sexual relationship with caution. In contrast, for Sigurd, a 35-year-old queer man also on PrEP, declaring one's PrEP status on Grindr signals an interest in condomless anal sex, which he does not associate with taking responsibility for one's own sexual health. He explains:

> If you meet someone on Grindr, they may write on their profile that they are on PrEP. It is good thing because it suggests that PrEP is not so stigmatised within this group of queer men. It is rare I speak to someone on Grindr who is on PrEP but does not declare it on their profile. When I do, I wonder why they do not declare it. There have been periods where I removed my PrEP status from Grindr, because I did not want people to assume that I was OK with condomless anal sex. (Sigurd, age 35, PrEP user)

For Sigurd, PrEP signals not only an interest in condomless anal sex, but also a vulnerability to sexually transmitted infection. Sigurd also indicates that it can be difficult to negotiate condom use if his Grindr profile shows that he is on PrEP. Similarly, Christian, a 26-year-old queer man on PrEP, details his experiences of unsuccessfully negotiating condom use with another PrEP user (see Figure 5.2):

> I want to share this photo to explain some of the experiences I have had with people on Grindr. One evening I was chatting with a guy, and we were planning to meet for sex. During the chat we started discussing protection. We were both on PrEP, but for him it was a deal-breaker if I was to insist on using condoms. He explained why

he did not want to use condoms. I occasionally have sex without condoms, but if condomless sex is a must for the other guy, I tend to say 'no thanks' myself. I feel I put myself at too high a risk of catching a sexually transmitted infection. I feel I have these discussions more and more often. (Christian, age 26, PrEP user)

For Christian and Klaus, PrEP represents two different things, both of which become visible and necessitate negotiation when chatting to other queer guys on dating apps like Grindr. According to Christian, these everyday negotiations

Figure 5.2: Rejected by people on PrEP

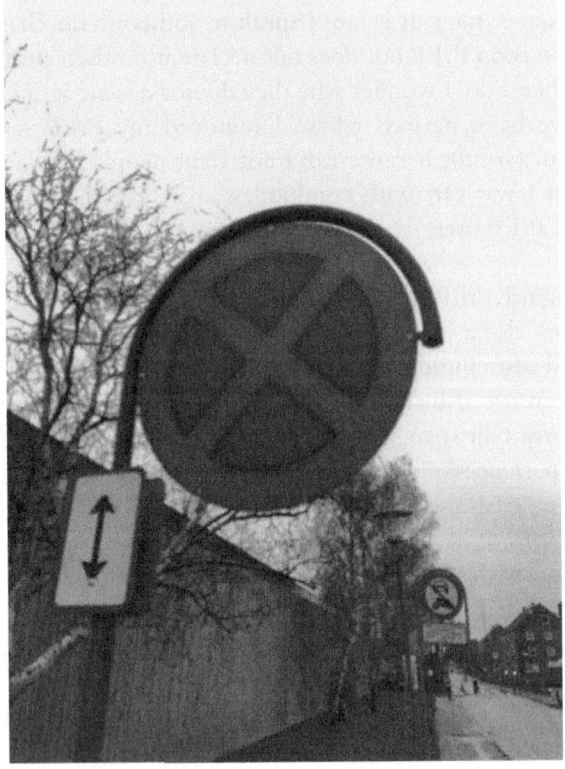

are happening more and more often. For Klaus, PrEP simply signals taking responsibility for preventing HIV, whereas for Sigurd and Christian, PrEP signals *both* responsibility for HIV prevention *and* irresponsibility by being associated with condomless anal sex and an increased likelihood of contracting a sexually transmitted infection. For queer men among whom taking PrEP is unambiguously considered a responsible thing to do, catching a sexually transmitted infection is not a major concern. It is 'just like catching a cold', as described by one participant; something that is quickly dealt with as part of their PrEP hospital controls. Still, for queer men in this 'camp', there is such a thing as catching too many sexually transmitted infections, as explained by Feng, and this is where ideas about 'irresponsible behaviour' and ambiguity can begin to sneak in:

> Within a period of eight months from September 2020 to April 2021, I contracted a sexually transmitted infection four times, plus corona [COVID-19]. Therefore, frequent check-ups were necessary. I was in Bispebjerg hospital multiple times. And I regretted my irresponsible behaviour on my own health. (Feng, age 35, PrEP user)

On the other hand, Sigurd, Christian, and others take PrEP more ambivalently, seeing it as being linked to both responsible and irresponsible sexual behaviour. Condom use, or lack thereof, and the potential for increases in other sexually transmitted infections play central roles in this fluctuation between linking PrEP to responsible or irresponsible sexual behaviour. This is clearly described by Mike, another PrEP user:

> People on PrEP take responsibility for themselves. And I think that's cool when people do. But it's clear that if I just fool around without a condom and don't think about whether I have chlamydia for example, then I wouldn't think it was very responsible, right? (Mike, age 32, PrEP user)

Another PrEP user, Stefan, takes the consideration of sexually transmitted infections to a whole other level, reflecting with guilt and uncertainty on the implications of condomless anal sex. Through questions, Stefan highlights some of the contentions, uncertainties, dilemmas, and ambiguities that he and his friends are dialectically considering:

> My friends [on PrEP] and I have the same considerations. How do we avoid transmission of sexually transmitted infections? Do we risk creating more resistant types of gonorrhea? Will we see new sexually transmitted infections? Are we selfish? I mean, are we a risk, a societal risk? Uh, come on out and spread some resistant bacteria through condomless sex. (Stefan, age 35, PrEP user)

What Stefan importantly highlights – by referring to his friends – is that different ideas and beliefs about condom use and the chances of contracting sexually transmitted infections are discussed differently across various social networks. This leads to varying norms and attitudes that may influence how these men interpret and prioritise the advice given by PrEP providers. Some men, like Sigurd and Mike, try to follow advice from healthcare workers to continue using condoms as much as possible, whereas other men place greater emphasis on the monitoring of sexually transmitted infections and accept that contracting gonorrhoea, syphilis, or chlamydia is part of the game. These different ideas often meet and collide during chats on dating apps like Grindr, necessitating negotiation and consideration. Worryingly, these different ideas may give rise to social divisions within the queer community, paradoxically alluding to an entirely different dimension of irresponsibility, with Klaus 'othering' non-PrEP users as being 'unsafe', and Sigurd expressing a slight frustration about his PrEP-peers' carelessness about other sexually transmitted infections and insistence on condomless anal sex.

I will return to the processes of 'othering' non-PrEP users later in this chapter. Meanwhile, I wish to end this section and irresponsible for having had unprotected sex with multiple sexual partners and for qualifying for PrEP. The queer men spoke highly about the healthcare staff who deliver PrEP, calling them non-judgemental. The shame thus came from comparing their sexual behaviour with ideas about 'good' or 'normal' sexual behaviour. Mike clarified the link between shame and 'deviance' from norms and ideas about 'good' sexual behaviour, and in the process highlighted how such feelings of shame may deter some people from accessing PrEP:

> To be considered eligible requires me to account for my sex life. Occurrences of condomless sex, sexually transmitted infections, et cetera. This makes PrEP inaccessible. To share the most intimate details of your life is scary. It takes a certain person to do that. I have worked hard not to be ashamed. We live in a culture where people get stigmatised for being sexually adventurous. It is called 'slut-shaming' and I fear this prevents people from accessing PrEP. People don't have the strength to disclose such details. They don't want to feel shame or be shamed for their desires or the choices they make. (Mike, age 32, PrEP user)

Unlike Sigurd, Mike did not talk about his own feelings of shame. He recognised the presence of shame in other people and explained that he has been on a journey of mental work to not be ashamed. He said that 'it takes a certain person' to unashamedly talk about one's sex life in a culture that judges and 'slut-shames' PrEP users. Later in our interview with Mike, he began to unpack what has helped him overcome the shame associated with PrEP use (and become this 'certain person'). When asked about how PrEP features in his friendship group, he explained:

> Not everyone is on PrEP, but relatively many are, and it's something we talk about. So, I know which of my friends

are on PrEP. It's normal in that sense, and nobody feels they are being shamed for being on PrEP. Or any longer, that is. There was a time, in the beginning, when people started using PrEP, where PrEP users were considered promiscuous. Now the tone is much, much nicer. Now taking PrEP is more about health and protecting yourself. And this has been normalised. There used to be an ugly tone, and some conversations were uncomfortable, but now we're more open, and it's nicer to talk about it. (Mike, age 32, PrEP user)

Mike navigates within a social network where PrEP is increasingly used and talked about, and where the members of his social network, through everyday PrEP negotiations, have shifted the narrative about PrEP from being related to irresponsible and promiscuous behaviour, to one characterised by taking responsibility for their health. His account of the change he has observed highlights the important role of informal networks in formulating opportunities for dialogue and creating new norms that help queer men 'get ahead' in relation to PrEP uptake. Sigurd also acknowledges the comfort he finds from having friends with whom he can talk about PrEP, captured through a photograph he took (see Figure 5.3):

I'm sharing this picture to illustrate that it's nice to have friends to talk about PrEP with (over a pink rim job cocktail!). We both started on PrEP at the same time, and it makes it easier when you can exchange experiences. Some people think 'you should just use a condom', so it's nice to have friends who are on the same page as yourself. (Sigurd, age 35, PrEP user)

PrEP is, for many queer men, an unwelcome reminder of so-called irresponsibilities, leading to feelings of shame. Queer friends and social networks were described as playing a pivotal role in finding comfort and reshaping this narrative. However,

Figure 5.3: Talking to friends

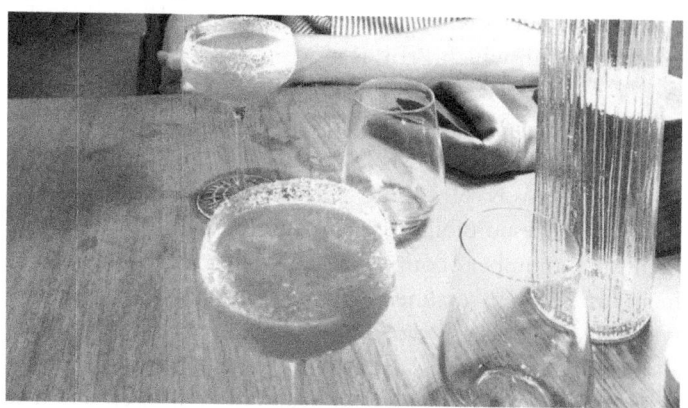

for a number of our queer participants, PrEP did not add to or remind them of shame. On the contrary: PrEP was said to remove shame altogether. It did so by eliminating the 'irresponsibility' of HIV risk arising from condomless queer sex. For this small group of queer men, HIV risk and related stigma were intrinsically linked to their sexuality and identity as queer men. By removing the risk of HIV from their sexuality, PrEP also removed shame from having sex with other men, as described by Toke:

> When I got onto PrEP I began to realise how ashamed I had been of my sexual behaviour. I realised that the shame I felt was connected to the risk of HIV. I struggled to come out as a gay man, I think because of this risk. With time, and when I got onto PrEP, I began to be at ease with my sexuality. Before I felt ashamed when having sex with another man. When I got onto PrEP, and the risk of HIV was eliminated, I began to feel much less shame. (Toke, age 27, PrEP user)

Although Toke had a different interpretation and experience from many of our other queer participants, he further underlines the deep-rooted hang-ups and shame associated with HIV, queer sex, and deviance from sexual norms in the context within which PrEP is used.

Am *I* irresponsible? 'Othering' non-PrEP users

Perhaps as a way of coping with negative stereotypes and notions of 'irresponsibility', and to develop more positive social identities, a number of our participants talked about themselves in an 'us' vs 'them' manner. Oftentimes, sentences that began with 'we, PrEP users' were followed by favourable statements about PrEP users and less flattering statements about non-PrEP users. For instance, Stefan, a 35-year-old PrEP user, said that in his social network of PrEP users, 'There is the prejudice that people who are not on PrEP are a little boring', with 'boring' referring to the notion of non-PrEP users as sexually less adventurous. This is supported by Mikkel, a 26-year-old PrEP user, who also demarcated clear boundaries between PrEP users and non-PrEP users, recognising that 'It's probably just a prejudice.' Mikkel describes how there are two types of gays: those who use apps like Grindr and those who do not; those who cruise and use saunas and those who do not. According to Mikkel, it is the former group that is on PrEP, and the group he favourably sees himself as being part of. For Mikkel, being on PrEP is a statement, signalling a rejection of the 'traditional' life. He explains: 'To have several sexual partners can be a type of statement. I don't aspire to a traditional life, or go out to look for a stable partner, someone to marry.'

Oral PrEP is not merely about taking a pill for HIV prevention. PrEP plays an integral role in forming social identities around PrEP use and in some social networks comes with the status of being adventurous and sexually liberated, as opposed to traditional and boring. Forming social identities around their adventurous and liberated sexualities not only helps PrEP users cope with 'slut-shaming', but also recasts the idea of 'being slutty' as something positive. Furthermore, and as alluded to earlier, many queer men were able to reconcile being sexually adventurous with being responsible. However, in the process of representing themselves as 'responsible' citizens preventing the spread of HIV, some inadvertently further reinforced the 'othering' of non-PrEP users, representing them as irresponsible. For instance, Bo, when discussing the need for PrEP to be made more easily accessible, explained that 'PrEP should be made more easily accessible for those who are not so good at taking responsibility for themselves.' As discussed earlier, this 'othering' occurs against the backdrop of recognising the limits of condom use. This 'othering' is thus conditional on practising safe sex. Mike explains: 'It is not that I think that people who are not on PrEP are irresponsible, as long as they use protection and go and get tested.' Similarly, Toke, without using the word 'irresponsible', describes how he would negatively view a non-PrEP user engaging in condomless anal sex:

> If he was very sexually active, and aware of PrEP, then I think it would, one way or the other, leave a negative impression [on me]. I would be thinking: Why on earth are you not protecting yourself, when you know that you have condomless sex, and know that this drug can eliminate the risk of HIV? (Toke, age 27, PrEP user)

Both Toke and Mike do not seek to 'other' queer men who are in monogamous relationships or able to consistently use condoms. They do, however, 'other' those men who are eligible for oral PrEP yet not enrolled.

The young women on PrEP in Zimbabwe did not explicitly 'other' women not using PrEP. They were generally understanding of the different challenges women face in accessing and using PrEP. However, when asked how they differed from non-PrEP-using women who are vulnerable to HIV, they often pointed to individual qualities. This included their ability to take control of and responsibility for their own potential PrEP users had to negotiate and manage stigma online, and that some managed to deal with blame and shame through a creative reappropriation of negative labels.

How queer men negotiate PrEP in everyday life is thus, to a large degree, influenced by how PrEP is talked about within their social networks. Consequently, social networks play a key role in determining how queer men navigate different understandings of what responsibility means in the context of PrEP, deal with feelings of shame, or demarcate differences between PrEP users and non-PrEP users. According to our research, such everyday PrEP negotiations play a defining role in queer men's experiences and continued engagement with PrEP in Denmark.

SIX

Healthy, yet a patient

This chapter covers the fourth paradox addressed in this book, namely that PrEP users are *both* healthy *and* patients. I alluded to this paradox in the opening paragraph of this book. All participants considered themselves healthy, and participants on PrEP had undergone careful screening to confirm their sexual health. Yet, despite being and considering themselves healthy, they also had to make sense of the need to adopt a patient persona centred around the PrEP treatment. The juxtaposition of having to prove one's good health and enrolling onto a medical treatment programme was stark and appears to be significant both for queer men in Denmark and young women in Zimbabwe, albeit with manifest differences, from various origins. This chapter shows how PrEP users, and those intending to use PrEP, work to reconcile and make sense of both being healthy and having to adopt the persona of a patient. For young women in Zimbabwe, such everyday PrEP negotiations happen against a background of living in a context where preventive pill-taking is met by scepticism and resistance, not least given the perceptions of PrEP side effects, and where treatment for HIV is common. For queer men in Denmark, the close monitoring of PrEP through selected infectious disease hospital departments appears to heighten the feeling of being a patient, and consequently, as a healthy person, the need to make sense of this.

The everyday PrEP negotiations arising from encountering ideas about being both healthy and a patient will be discussed under three headings capturing core deliberations and negotiation work:

- What am I treating when I am not sick? Difficulties reconciling the 'patient' persona with being healthy
- How do I give meaning to the PrEP treatment? Rethinking PrEP as a treatment to maintain health
- Is it worth it? Weighing up the preventive potential against side effects and HIV

What am I treating when I am not sick? Difficulties reconciling the 'patient' persona with being healthy

Both young women in Zimbabwe and queer men in Denmark described having difficulties reconciling their good health with the need to adopt the persona of a patient and to comply with the therapy offered. Descriptions of this tension differed slightly between the two settings, partly explained by cultural norms around pill-taking for prevention. For young women in Zimbabwe, for instance, discussions of the dissonance between being 'healthy, yet a patient' centred around the strangeness of pill-taking for prevention. Ashley, who is on PrEP herself, alludes to what she describes as a common notion in her community, namely that taking an HIV prevention pill is an absurd thing to do. As Erisy further describes, this so-called absurdity lies in the paradoxical nature of being healthy yet required to be on treatment:

> For now, people think it's absurd to take the medication [PrEP] for HIV prevention. But taking a pill for prevention is better than taking a pill for HIV treatment. (Ashley, age 25, on PrEP)

> Most people shun the idea of taking tablets when not sick. They ask questions like, 'What am I treating when I'm not sick?' It's this kind of mentality that makes people decide against the use of PrEP and go for condoms instead. (Erisy, age 24, eligible for PrEP)

Both Ashley and Erisy capture the shared cultural belief and attitude that pill-taking is merely for treating illness and that this idea may obstruct PrEP uptake. However, Erisy also demonstrates that it is possible to approach pill-taking as a form of health maintenance – an idea I explore in detail in the next section. Queer men in Denmark also often mentioned pill-taking as something they associate with illness. This is captured by Jens, who is interested in PrEP but filled with ambivalence:

> Medicine and pills have never been my cup of tea. What am I swallowing? What does it do to my body and mind, here and now and in the future? I don't take pills if my gums hurt after a visit to the dentist, if I'm hungover, or if I'm feeling unwell. I eat well, sleep well and exercise regularly. This makes me feel healthy. For me, pills like those in the picture (see Figure 6.1) represent illnesses that put limits on my daily life and freedom. It's precisely such feelings that PrEP speaks to. But, do they improve my daily life? Do they provide me with more freedom? Yes. Unequivocally, yes. (Jens, age 40, PrEP interested)

The ambivalence expressed by Jens revolves around his difficulties in reconciling the perceived benefits of PrEP against a broader scepticism about medication. For Jens, the tension lies between his general resistance to pills – which he portrays as symbols of illness and limitation – and the specific recognition that PrEP is an exception, offering tangible improvements to his daily life and levels of freedom. What Ashley, Erisy, and Jens capture is the duality of complex and conflictual ideas that

Figure 6.1: Pills, more pills

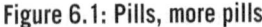

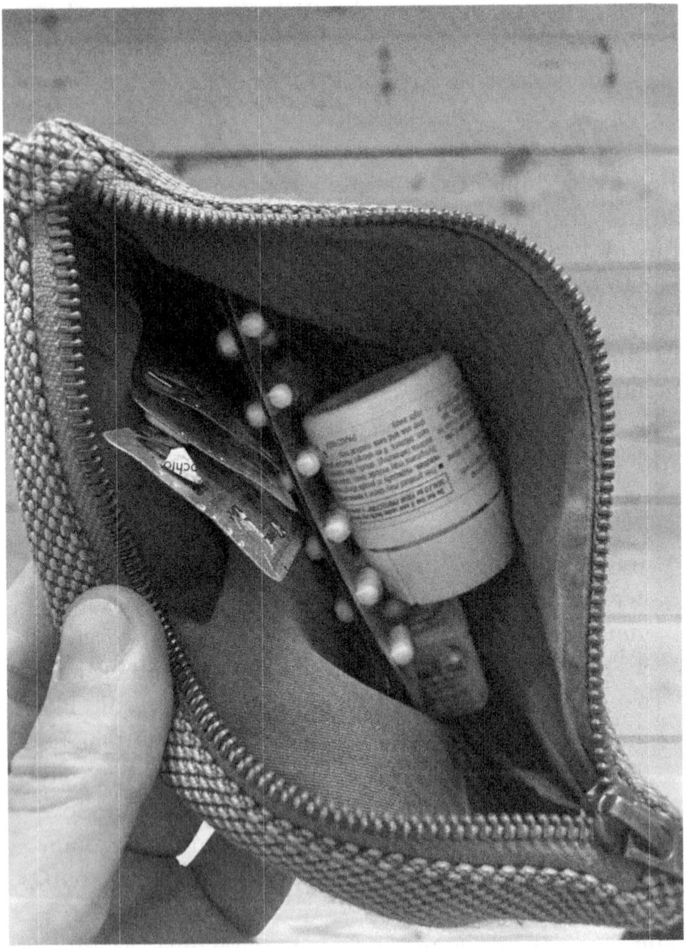

people either using or interested in PrEP must negotiate and give meaning to in day-to-day life.

For queer men on PrEP, however, the whole experience of going to an infectious disease department at a hospital for eligibility screening and getting enrolled on PrEP was emphasised by some as being particularly difficult to reconcile

Figure 6.2: The hospital

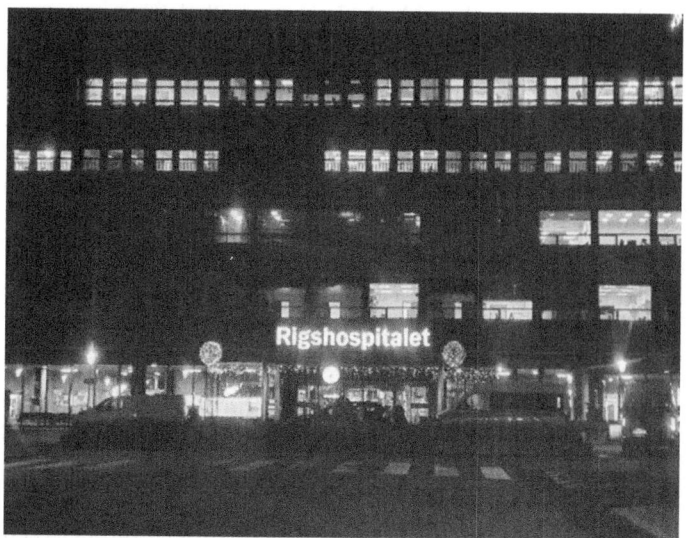

with being healthy. They described the hospital-based PrEP service in Denmark as 'overwhelming' and 'extreme', a process that pathologises the individual and 'makes you feel sick'. Much of this was captured by Poul, who describes his ambivalence with being healthy while at the same time being enrolled in a hospital-based treatment programme (see Figure 6.2):

> Throughout my life, I've been to the hospital maybe two to three times. Now I must go there every three months to get checked. In a way, it's overwhelming, and having to take pills regularly falls into the same category. There is a special atmosphere in a hospital. Whether you're sick or not, I find that I get sicker or feel sick when I am in a hospital. That way, I feel like a sick person going to check for a serious illness. And I associate the hospital with two opposites: life that begins and life that ends. (Poul, age 46, PrEP user)

The juxtaposition of having virtually no contact with the health services and suddenly being enrolled in a treatment programme that requires regular check-ups at hospital-based infectious disease departments was stark for many of our queer participants, not least because they associated the hospital space with the treatment of severe illness. This both made some of them feel sick and amplified their sense of patienthood.

This section has highlighted a tension between maintaining a sense of health and the necessity of adopting a 'patient' persona for therapeutic compliance. For young women in Zimbabwe, the perceived absurdity associated with pill-taking despite being in good health underscores a prevailing idea that links pill consumption exclusively to the treatment of illness. In this cultural context, this shared understanding can become a significant impediment to widespread PrEP use. For queer men in Denmark, ideas of PrEP services as rigid and hospital-centric, coupled with associations between the hospital environment and serious illness, magnified their sense of patienthood. The next section will further explore how individuals respond to difficulties in reconciling the 'patient' persona with being healthy, focusing on their efforts to challenge the pathologising of PrEP and to redefine pill-taking as a form of health maintenance, as opposed to a response to illness.

How do I give meaning to the PrEP treatment? Rethinking PrEP as a treatment to maintain health

Our participants responded in different ways to the paradox of being both healthy and required to adopt a 'patient' persona. However, what they share is a broad commitment to downplaying the patienthood associated with PrEP treatment, and instead rethinking PrEP as a health-maintaining activity. For queer men, this involved creating a distance between their daily normal and healthy selves and the pathologising of their infectious disease risk and treatment of their 'sick' sexuality. This brings me back to Chapter 4, where I argued that PrEP is primarily administered as a public health good, meaning national health services make it available for free to prevent infectious disease risk, and target so-called high-risk groups in the most cost-effective way. While this makes sense from a health economics and health administrator perspective, Chapter 4 noted that rigid screening procedures and controls to identify and treat those demonstrating past vulnerabilities to HIV do not necessarily resonate with what queer men think should be criteria for PrEP eligibility. Consequently, to be eligible to be prescribed PrEP, some queer men applied – with unease – their own sexual health-promoting and future-oriented eligibility criteria. The paradox discussed in this chapter further illuminates this contention.

Mike, a 32-year-old PrEP user in Denmark, ties together many of the themes discussed in the book thus far in his description of a photograph of his local pharmacy (see Figure 6.3). For Mike and others, the pharmacy is an unwelcome reminder of the seriousness, rigidity, and control of their PrEP treatment, and by extension, their sense of patienthood. Mike explains why:

> This photo is a picture of my local pharmacy. Here, I can't obtain my medication like people with chronic illnesses can. My medication is not on prescription, my name is not on it. To get my medication, I have to go to the hospital and undergo tests and examinations – and I have to be approved for it. Approval that requires me to account for my sex life, how many I've had unprotected sex with, whether I've had sexually transmitted diseases, and more. And that makes PrEP inaccessible. Having to disclose the most intimate parts of your life is frightening. It takes a toll [on you] to expose yourself like that. Especially a part of my life that I've had to fight not to be ashamed of – because we grow up in a culture where people are stigmatised for believing in free love. It's called

'slut-shaming' – and I fear that both young and old will opt out of PrEP because they can't handle revealing themselves and details about the most intimate parts of their lives, as they don't want to feel shame or be made to feel ashamed of their desires or the choices they make. (Mike, age 32, PrEP user)

Mike's strategy to make sense of the paradox of being 'healthy, yet a patient' is to critically examine the circumstances that require him to adopt the persona of a patient. In describing another photograph, Mike goes on to explain how being a 'patient', and having PrEP reduced to a public health good, makes him feel:

I'm a statistic. A group of health professionals follow me. They comply with guidelines on eligibility, dispensing practices and control follow-up with the aim of making my treatment cost-effective. Despite meeting good, skilled and understanding nurses and doctors, I often feel that I'm part of a system, an object, rather than a human being. (Mike, age 32, PrEP user)

Mike clearly articulates his feeling of being reduced to a number, or an object whose sexuality needs to be controlled and treated in the most cost-effective way. Not all our

Figure 6.3: The pharmacy

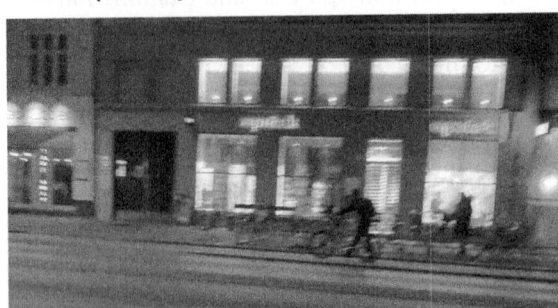

participants were as articulate or as critical as Mike, but they nonetheless spoke to a rejection of PrEP as merely a public health good. Similar to what was discussed in Chapter 4, queer PrEP users, in an attempt to distance themselves from the patienthood cast upon them by the hospital-centric PrEP treatment programme, reframed PrEP as a form of self-care and health maintenance. PrEP was regularly compared to annual vaccines or vitamin pills – something you get or take to protect and maintain health, as described by Mike and Bo:

> I see it [PrEP] as getting an annual flu vaccine, only that I take the medicine daily. Fundamentally, I approach PrEP as a health maintaining thing. (Mike, age 32, PrEP user)

> I've compared it [PrEP] a lot to taking a vitamin pill. I mean. After all, it's also taking a pill. I don't take it because I'm sick. I think I'm comparing PrEP quite a lot to the fact that it's preventive – to take better care of yourself. It's not because you're sick. It's because you can get sick. Kind of like getting to it in advance. So, I see it more as a vitamin pill. (Bo, age 21, PrEP experienced)

Feng also talked about how he had embedded his PrEP pill-taking into other daily health management practices, stating, 'PrEP is just a daily pill I take together with all my vitamin pills.' By drawing parallels with routine preventive measures, such as getting a non-mandatory flu vaccine or taking vitamin pills, Mike, Bo, and Feng shift the narrative away from a focus on concrete infectious disease risk and the treatment of their 'unconventional sexual behaviour', to one centred on health maintenance and the more diffuse and hard-to-see vulnerabilities that come with a happy and healthy sex life.

Young women in Zimbabwe also recast PrEP as a treatment to maintain health, self-care, and well-being. However, partly due to Zimbabwe's more flexible PrEP services, and the fact that their sexuality is not the subject of public health control in the same way as it is experienced by queer men in Denmark, they did not do so from the perspective of feeling pathologised. On the contrary, they often spoke about their husbands' uncontrollable sexuality, revealing a collective understanding that men are often unfaithful to their wives and refuse to use condoms. These ideas are captured by Ashley, who argues that PrEP is a way for her to care for herself, given her chances of contracting HIV from her husband:

> I learned and understood what PrEP is and decided to use it because, to be honest, no man is faithful. They will always have sex out there and may not use protection, hence putting me at risk. So, taking PrEP will help reduce the chances of being infected by the virus regardless of my husband's behaviour. (Ashley, age 25, PrEP experienced)

Many young women explained the value of PrEP from this perspective, with the anticipation of their male partner's HIV risk generally being considered a motivating factor for their own sustained PrEP use, as described by 23-year-old Angela, who is on PrEP: 'I was thinking of stopping taking the pills then, but I then thought "What if my husband is engaging in risky sexual behaviour out there?" so it made me continue to take PrEP.' Later in our interview with Angela, she detailed the importance of being able to reduce the likelihood of contracting HIV. In one of our focus group discussions with the young women, the discussion at some point focused on how PrEP would enable them, as women, to put themselves first, giving them peace of mind. In this sense, enrolling in PrEP treatment is considered pivotal to self-care. Maidei expands on this idea in her description of how PrEP is key to maintaining health and being able to live a productive life, being able to sustain oneself and not rely on one's husband:

> Therefore, for [some]one to be able to make money, there is a certain level of health they are supposed to have to

ensure that they can work for themselves. The desire to work and make your own money would encourage you to take up PrEP to ensure that you're healthy and not at risk of getting HIV. (Maidei, age 26, eligible for PrEP)

The need for young women to be able to reduce their vulnerabilities to HIV, as well as their dependency on men was omnipresent in our Zimbabwe data. Young women on PrEP communicated this need not only to the interviewer, but also to each other, as described by Stella, a 26-year-old PrEP user: 'When we talk, we always remind each other of the reason why we are taking these pills in the first place.' This 'reminding' not only supports engagement with PrEP, but also reproduces many of the ideas outlined earlier, reframing PrEP as a form of self-care.

As our participants make sense of PrEP, and the paradox that they are healthy, yet need to take a daily pill and be subject to a strict treatment regime, they contemplate what PrEP offers them. In so doing, they reveal a widening discrepancy between how PrEP users understand and experience PrEP as a medication that on the one hand positively promotes and maintains health in the broadest sense, and on the other is associated with pathology because of the way PrEP services are delivered as a form of public health good, with a narrow focus on population risk and prevention of infectious disease, rather than on self-care. This tension appears more pronounced among queer men in Denmark, where PrEP services are more rigid and the subject of treatment is the queer men's own sexuality.

Is it worth it? Weighing up the preventive potential against side effects and HIV

Up to this point, the chapter has centred on a duality arising from the paradox 'healthy, yet a patient'. On the one hand, PrEP necessitates a 'patient' persona and triggers associations with treatment for illness. On the other hand, and in response to the former, there is the counterbalancing notion that PrEP promotes self-care and serves as a form of health maintenance. This section introduces a different dilemma, namely ambivalence arising from ideas and ways of thinking that – in the context of treatment availability – make you begin to question the worth and value of PrEP if it leaves you sick from side effects and you become an actual patient.

Side effects from PrEP were talked about as minimal among our PrEP-using participants. Several young women on PrEP mentioned experiencing slight side effects for a couple of days after starting PrEP or if they swallowed the pill without eating first, but that was all. However, for young PrEP-inexperienced women, the anticipated side effects affected their perceptions of PrEP and played a contributing role in their decision not to take it up. Many of the PrEP-inexperienced women we spoke to asked the interviewer not *if* but *what* side effects come with PrEP, demonstrating both their concerns about and assumption of anticipated side effects, and their lack of concrete knowledge. Alison and Stephanie both described the prevailing idea that PrEP is associated with anticipated side effects:

> People think that PrEP has some side effects, and that's when some will start discouraging women from accessing PrEP and not taking the pills. (Alison, age 21, eligible for PrEP)

> Many women do not understand that PrEP does not have side effects. Many people think that the tablet will make you fat, and some are saying you will have a headache. People are saying a lot of things. (Stephanie, age 23, PrEP user)

The mention of concerns about weight gain and headaches reflects a social representation circulating within the community about some of the anticipated adverse effects of PrEP. These effects may, as alluded to by Alison, outweigh the perceived benefits of PrEP. Precious delves into some of the reasons why anticipated side effects matter so much:

> My husband knows some tablets may cause weight gain, headaches and other things. Let's say I start taking the pill today, and after three months, my husband sees me gaining weight or losing weight. He will ask me, 'What's going on?' He will start questioning me and being suspicious. (Precious, age 22, eligible for PrEP)

Precious highlights that side effects are not merely an individual experience, but are intertwined with social dynamics. Ideas about anticipated side effects and the perceived manifestation of these influence how PrEP itself is perceived, discussed, and accepted or rejected by individuals within the community, or indeed within relationships. Ideas about the anticipated side effects of pill-taking must be considered against the background of the scaling up of antiretroviral therapy for HIV treatment. In this context, most people will know someone living with HIV and on treatment, or will have heard about side effects from antiretroviral pill-taking. As PrEP is also an antiretroviral drug, the cross-fertilisation of ideas and beliefs about anticipated side effects may create a grey zone in which a husband may accuse his wife of taking antiretroviral drugs either for treatment or prevention of HIV, because he sees her as not trusting him to be sexually faithful to her.

Another reason to consider PrEP in the context of antiretroviral therapy is the belief that taking antiretroviral pills for treatment makes more sense than taking pills for prevention. In a focus group discussion with young women eligible for PrEP, Maria highlighted the idea that young people are not particularly concerned about contracting HIV and then taking antiretroviral pills for treatment, also given the 'absurdity' of pill-taking as discussed earlier: 'Young people will start questioning themselves, saying, why should they take PrEP pills every day knowing that they are not sick? People don't care about that; they will prefer to take the ARV pills after testing HIV positive.'

This idea was also raised by two queer men in Denmark. The quality of antiretroviral therapy, coupled with a low-risk perception, meant that some queer men began to question the relevance of PrEP. This was described by Poul in one of his Photovoice stories (see Figure 6.4):

> I am considering dropping out of the PrEP programme. I feel sick when I take them. They're not necessary, like a vaccine that's supposed to reduce significant infection rates. The incidence rates of HIV are low, particularly among the age groups I sleep with. If I were to acquire HIV, it wouldn't be such a big deal. The only challenge would be taking the daily pill again. (Poul, age 46, PrEP user)

Poul is weighing up the benefits of PrEP against the chances and consequences of contracting HIV. Because of his

Figure 6.4: Pills

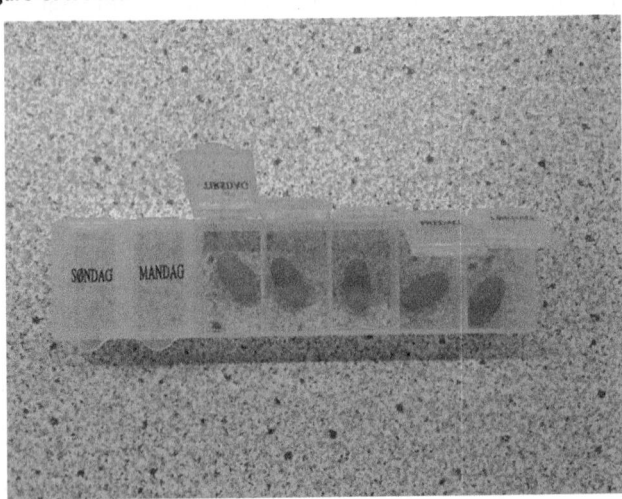

ambivalent feelings, he is still considering this. Mikkel is also contemplating the value of PrEP, and he is unsure if the work associated with PrEP patienthood balances the likelihood of contracting HIV:

> It's a lot *of* work. You need to remember to take the pill every day to be certain that you are protected. I've never really liked taking pills, and all of a sudden, I'm taking a daily pill without being ill, and to prevent something I only have a small chance of contracting HIV. If there was a 50% chance of getting infected, or something like that, it would make more sense to be on PrEP. It seems like a lot of hassle. (Mikkel, age 26, PrEP user)

This section has shown that a multifaceted system of values, ideas, and beliefs can result in uncertainty and ambiguity concerning the value of PrEP. The ambivalence appears to stem from the perceived worth and work involved with being a PrEP 'patient', weighed against anticipated side effects, the availability of HIV treatment, and the perception of HIV vulnerability.

Conclusion

What am I treating when I am not sick? How do I give meaning to PrEP treatment? Is it worth it? These questions capture core deliberations and reflections that underpin some of the everyday PrEP negotiations that arise from PrEP users having to navigate the dual representation of being *both* healthy individuals *and* patients. Building on findings presented in Chapter 4, the deliberations reveal some fundamental rifts between how oral PrEP is delivered as a public health good that aims to cost-effectively prevent the spread of HIV in so-called high-risk groups, and the ways in which individuals make sense of and integrate PrEP into their lives.

SEVEN

Safe, yet unsafe

The fifth and penultimate paradox covered in this book relates to how PrEP *both* keeps its users safe from HIV infection *and* introduces new elements of unsafety. This paradox manifests itself very differently between the study contexts and to varying degrees between the participants. However, what all study participants share is a collective trust in PrEP's ability to prevent the acquisition of HIV when exposed to the virus. At no point in our two studies did a participant question the efficacy of PrEP. However, in as much as PrEP was represented as a safety net in the context of HIV vulnerability, it was also associated with other risks and harm. For young women in Zimbabwe, this related to shared understandings of the risks of violence, abuse, and abandonment from parents or partners if it was discovered they were on PrEP. For queer men in Denmark, it related primarily to two different issues. For some, PrEP was linked to the amplification of more potentially harmful sexual practices, such as using drugs as part of their sex life – a phenomenon also known as chemsex. For others, the unknown and potentially negative long-term health impacts of PrEP were disconcerting.

The dialectics arising from opposing ideas about PrEP being both safe and unsafe brought about different deliberations and everyday PrEP negotiations. These will be discussed under the following headings:

- What social risks come with oral PrEP? Weighing up the perceived dangers of PrEP protection against HIV
- Does taking PrEP impact my sexuality in a negative way? Ambivalences concerning how PrEP may augment harmful sexual practices
- Is PrEP safe in the long term? Concerns about the unknown long-term effects of PrEP

What social risks come with oral PrEP? Weighing up the perceived dangers of PrEP protection against HIV

As discussed in the previous chapter, young women spoke highly about oral PrEP and its ability to keep them safe from HIV, not least because of their husbands' infidelity and their own lack of power to negotiate condom use. However, in addition to this understanding, young women in Zimbabwe overwhelmingly referred to a shared belief that PrEP is associated with unsafety in the form of social risks from PrEP use. More specifically and reflecting the cultural and patriarchal context of eastern Zimbabwe, young women spoke lucidly about the incompatibility of PrEP with the norms and values surrounding what it means to be a 'good girl'. PrEP signals intentions of having sex, which, in this cultural context, challenge prevailing gender norms and expectations of 'good girls' not to have sex before or outside of marriage. The idea that PrEP is incompatible with local understandings of 'good girls' was said to lead to different forms of social control, including stigma and discrimination, or even violence, abuse, and abandonment. The social control is enacted by parents, partners, healthcare workers, and the broader community. One adolescent girl (Patience) talked about how protecting herself from HIV through PrEP would 'raise wars' at home with her parents. She went on to say that 'this deters young people from wanting to use PrEP as a HIV prevention method'. Recognising the safety and protective potential of PrEP, Patience was keen for young women to take it up, but simultaneously accepted the shared belief that this may be unsafe from a social and relational perspective. Many young women also spoke about the physical violence they could face from their male partner if they took oral PrEP secretly and without his approval. Maria and Angela explained:

> He will start wondering what those pills are for. You will face abuse from your partner. He will ask you what those pills are for and if you fail to explain everything to him, you will end up getting beaten up for that. (Maria, age 18–24, eligible for PrEP)

> Their spouses will be offended if they find out that their wives want to be on PrEP and this may result in domestic violence. (Angela, age 23, PrEP user)

Most young women in our study ascribed to the idea that parents and partners would disapprove of their PrEP use, even when they themselves had experienced the opposite. Take Angela as an example. A key element of her own ability to use PrEP has been having an open dialogue with her husband. But despite her own experiences, she recognised and reproduced the idea that most parents or partners would disapprove of PrEP, and described the potential risks involved with young women taking PrEP behind their husband's backs:

> What makes me different is that my husband and I communicate well and freely. Many other women are unable to do that. They may want to take PrEP in secret, without their spouses' knowledge. However, this may be problematic if the husband were to find out and this could lead to domestic violence. (Angela, age 23, PrEP user)

Other women spoke about the risk of being abandoned by their husbands if the men discovered their PrEP use. Much more can be said about how social representations of 'good girls' in this cultural context come to shape different forms of social control, with implications for young women's PrEP use. I covered this in Chapters 3 and 4.

The social representation that PrEP might lead to 'wars' at home, violence, and abandonment has its roots in the gender orders that characterise the socio-cultural context of our study, and that are maintained through how young women talk about PrEP with each other, and indeed in interview situations like ours. Opposing ideas about the safety of PrEP leave young women with the difficult dilemma of having to weigh up the safety and protective potential of PrEP against the social risks of abuse and abandonment. PrEP may provide safety from contracting HIV and be accessible for free, but using it may also come at a very high social cost in the form of physical and psychosocial impacts and strained interpersonal relationships. This necessitates substantial everyday PrEP negotiations, both within the individual who has to make sense of and weigh up the safety and unsafety of PrEP in the context of their daily life, and also between young women and their partners, as well as between young women as they share their concerns with each other.

This section has exclusively focused on the social risks of PrEP use from the perspective of young women in Zimbabwe. However, as discussed in Chapter 5, queer men also face social risks in the form of 'slut-shaming' and judgement from people around them. While this may, for some, result in a similar dilemma of having to weigh up social risks against their chances of contracting HIV, for our queer participants this did not appear to be pivotal to their decision-making. That said, one of the co-researchers in the PrEPping project, a PrEP service provider, explained to me that several of her clients experienced internalised homophobia or were part of social networks in which stigma against the queer community is common. This stigma delayed and complicated their uptake of and engagement with PrEP.

Does taking PrEP impact my sexuality in a negative way? Ambivalences concerning how PrEP may augment harmful sexual practices

An issue that affected several queer men in Denmark, but was not evident in our data from young women in Zimbabwe, was the role of PrEP in amplifying more harmful sexual practices. Chapter 5 explored how PrEP is, for queer men, often linked to a more vibrant and active sex life – something many of them celebrate, yet also associate with more transmission of sexually transmitted infections.

Some of our queer participants also expressed growing anxiety about the connection between PrEP and chemsex. For a few of our participants, this was rooted in personal experience. Stefan, a 35-year-old PrEP user, remarked: 'I think that maybe it [PrEP] has influenced me to have sex [while] on drugs to a greater extent than I had before.'

Two of our queer participants expressed ambivalence about PrEP's growing association with chemsex. For both, PrEP has allowed them to enter sexual networks and subcultures within the queer community where chemsex is practised. Here they have found a non-judgemental community and enjoy practising chemsex, with PrEP protecting them against HIV. Yet they simultaneously articulate some of the dangers and problems associated with chemsex, as illustrated by Toke:

> Among some gay men, perhaps especially in Berlin, there is a kind of culture where it's just about doing what you feel like. Being with the people you want to be with. And where you celebrate autonomy or rebelliousness, and do not want to accept all the norms of society. There is a special culture very much centred around music and party and sex and, and drugs in some way. Um. Which I also have found joy in being a part of. But I can also

see a lot of problems with it. If you take a step back, you think: okay, it's just a lot of people who are running away from reality because they're not processing a lot of the things they're dealing with, right? (Toke, age 27, PrEP user)

Toke elevates the idea that PrEP helps liberate queer sex, which in some subcultures within the queer community may include chemsex. Toke expresses a tension between the sense of joy and liberation that comes with chemsex on the one hand, and acknowledgement of the downsides on the other, including potential problems and escapism from reality, which can be potentially harmful. Feng, a 35-year-old PrEP user who migrated to Denmark from East Asia, also has an ambivalent relationship with chemsex. Since he took up PrEP, Feng has been part of what he calls 'the bold and experimental gay community', which has taken his sexuality to a whole new level. Feng took a photograph of his PrEP medication box (see Figure 7.1), and in his description of the photograph he alludes to the representation of PrEP users as people who engage in chemsex:

Let's be honest, PrEP is taken by many people for unprotected sex. Sex workers might have a different agenda but for queer men the purposes are less glorious, if not sinister, with the indulgence of chemsex and group orgies. I began to have sex without protection as well. (Feng, age 35, PrEP user)

For Feng there is a strong association between PrEP use, chemsex, and an unsafe lifestyle. Feng has participated in multiple sex- and drug-filled parties and has found a community in this subculture. While Feng, like Toke, finds joy in this, he also, in different parts of the interview, expresses ambivalence and discomfort with the association between PrEP use and chemsex: 'It's not PrEP related, but um maybe it's a

Figure 7.1: PrEP and party and play

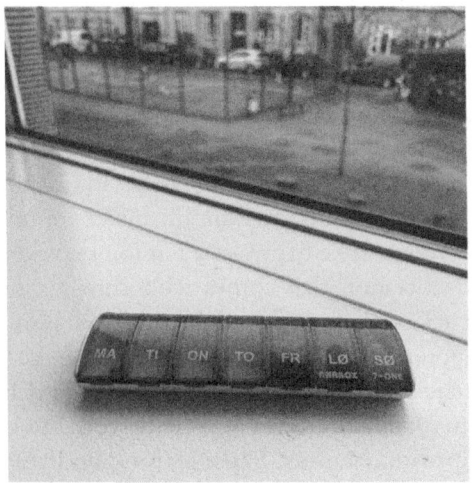

little bit PrEP related. But there's a tendency.' Feng goes on to talk about how his participation in drug-filled sex parties has led to him contracting multiple sexually transmitted infections (see Chapter 5), linking PrEP with what he calls irresponsible behaviour. He goes on to say, 'I will continue with PrEP in a more responsible manner.' Feng appreciates how PrEP has allowed him to engage in chemsex and form a strong social and sexual network, yet he feels uncomfortable and ambivalent about what PrEP use has come to mean to him, associating it with going beyond norms of safe sexual practices. This paradoxical tension and the related ambivalence form part of Feng's everyday PrEP negotiation, through which he weighs up the social benefits and joy he gets from chemsex against the health risks and discomfort of being a drug user.

Among some of our queer participants there is a prevailing idea that PrEP, due to its power to keep people safe from contracting HIV, enables them to venture into new sexual territories, which include chemsex. Chemsex is associated with risk. The risks may be small for some people, but are more harmful for others, with dependency, anxiety, and depression being some of the potential harmful impacts. The absence of accounts depicting responsible and low-risk chemsex practices, along with the identified ambivalences, indicate that the queer men in our study associate chemsex with risk and unsafety. Queer men within this context are compelled to navigate and negotiate the tensions inherent in the duality of the PrEP–chemsex relationship – balancing the joy, liberation, and sense of community it brings, while also acknowledging potential harm and discomfort stemming from PrEP and its evolving association with chemsex.

Is PrEP safe in the long term? Concerns about the unknown long-term effects of PrEP

When asked about concerns regarding PrEP, only a few participants expressed apprehension or uncertainty about its safety, indicating broad trust in the safety profile of PrEP as a pharmaceutical drug. When concerns were raised, they were often phrased as questions, reflecting uncertainty and a lack of knowledge in this area. Stephanie was the only young female participant who expressed uncertainty, and she did so through putting a question to the interviewer: 'Does the tablet have some after-effects after some years?' Among the queer men, Stefan also raised questions about the long-term safety of PrEP:

> What is this [referring to PrEP]? Could you be harmed by it? After seven to twelve months on PrEP, I stopped for thirty weeks because I was like, well, if I'm not going to have changing sex partners, maybe it's stupid for me to stay on PrEP. Can I be damaged by it? Is it safe for me to do this? Do we know enough about it [PrEP]? (Stefan, age 35, PrEP user)

Against a background of much uncertainty, Stefan is contemplating the safety aspects of PrEP. He is considering the possibility of PrEP having negative effects on his health, so much so that he weighs them up against his risk perception, affecting his continued engagement with PrEP. José's remarks indicate similar deliberations. But rather than discontinuing PrEP, he contemplates shifting from daily to 'on-demand' oral PrEP:

> When I first approached my medical provider, she informed me that I could take oral PrEP 'on demand' or daily. Since I decided that I didn't want to plan when to have sex, I incorporated the pill into my daily routine. This way I am ready to engage in sexual relations 'on the spot' without thinking about HIV that much. Sometimes I consider switching to 'on demand' because I don't want to put too much pressure on my kidneys and bones which are impacted by PrEP. Even though these effects may be limited, I still think about the long-term effects of PrEP, which I'm not aware of. (José, age 23, PrEP user)

As alluded to by José, often when PrEP safety was discussed, queer men referred to the shared and collective understanding that PrEP is harsh on their kidneys. This idea, as explained by both José and Klaus, has its origin in the initial eligibility screening process, where healthy kidneys are a criterion that is closely monitored:

> My initial concern was related to my kidneys because I know that you put some pressure on your kidneys when you start taking PrEP. PrEP services check your kidneys before you start treatment and I remember being really concerned about that because in my family my grandmother died from kidney failure. I have this thing in my head telling me that because of my family background, my kidneys are more likely to be affected. (José, age 23, PrEP user)

> I would like to become a father at some point, and I wonder if there are any long-term effects of PrEP that

may affect my fertility or whether it can damage the foetus. I don't know. Things like this have been quite important to me. I had been told that this medicine is harsh, harsh in the sense that it can affect the liver. This is also why they keep an eye on my liver numbers, whether they look okay. (Klaus, age 42, PrEP user)

What José and Klaus also exemplify is how particular circumstances, such as having a family history of poor kidneys or having a desire to become a father, can amplify concerns and attention around the safety of PrEP. Holic, who is 32 and on PrEP, mentioned in his interview how obtaining PrEP online – which he did prior to accessing PrEP from the national health services in Denmark – heightened his concerns about what he was consuming and the potential harm it was causing.

Concern and uncertainty about the long-term safety of PrEP was an issue raised by only a few participants, again, indicating broad and widespread trust in the safety profile of PrEP. Those who did raise concerns did so because of 'not knowing', or from the common understanding that PrEP negatively impacts the kidneys. Interestingly, they were all on PrEP. They trusted the safety profile of PrEP enough to be on it, perhaps swayed by its many benefits, yet they still expressed uncertainty and concerns about the long-term implications of PrEP use.

Conclusion

What social risks come with PrEP? Does taking PrEP impact my sexuality in a negative way? Is PrEP safe in the long term? These three questions capture some of the safety concerns and uncertainties that come with PrEP, despite an otherwise widespread trust in PrEP's safety profile and ability to keep people safe from contracting HIV if exposed. The findings presented in this chapter provide background on the origin of various safety concerns and detail everyday PrEP negotiations arising from PrEP being considered *both* safe *and* unsafe.

The nature of and need for PrEP negotiations because of uncertainty arising from PrEP's association with risks and harm differ significantly between queer men in Denmark and young women in Zimbabwe. However, for both groups, these negotiations are not made any easier by the recognition of the many benefits associated with PrEP.

In Zimbabwe, patriarchy and strong public gender norms introduce considerable safety concerns for young women. Previous chapters have noted how young women's disenfranchised position prevents them from having the financial means to access PrEP (Chapter 3), but not from having their eligibility questioned and challenged by people around them (Chapter 4). This chapter further emphasises these forces by detailing strong shared ideas about the social safety risks young women may face if they take up PrEP. Rooted in cultural understandings of what it means to be a 'good girl', there is a strong perceived lack of social acceptability, with shared assumptions about how parents or partners may react if the woman's PrEP use is discovered (Skovdal et al., 2022a). Importantly, young women on PrEP provide counter-examples of support, suggesting variations in social acceptability. Elsewhere, we have reported on parents' conflicting attitudes towards PrEP, with some expressing support for it (Skovdal et al., 2023). Using survey data, we have found a similar weakening of social norms, with almost universal recognition of young women having premarital sex and substantial support for making condoms available to teenage girls (Gregson et al., 2024). Nonetheless, despite the attenuation of negative public gender norms and mixed attitudes towards PrEP, the prevailing and shared belief that there is a widespread lack of social acceptability creates a background for everyday PrEP negotiations. Worries and fears of violence or abandonment present the dilemma of having to weigh up the perceived social risks of PrEP use with PrEP's potential to protect and keep them safe from HIV. In a context where there is a generally low-risk perception, many young women may err on the side of caution against social risks and choose not to take up PrEP (Skovdal et al., 2022a).

The safety concerns raised by queer men in Denmark did not appear to be an obstacle to their PrEP uptake. Instead, the safety concerns helped them reflect on how PrEP works on them and their bodies. Queer men do not just passively swallow PrEP pills, but continually evaluate PrEP's impact on their lives. For some, this involved ambivalent reflection on how PrEP was transforming their sex lives and serving as a gateway to more daring and risky sexual practices, such as chemsex. For others, it was about thinking through the unknown long-term impacts of PrEP use. In both examples, queer men attach potential harms and risks to PrEP use, which they subsequently juxtapose and weigh against PrEP's liberating and protective benefits. For some, such everyday PrEP negotiations may prevent them from falling victim to the harmful effects of chemsex, and for others, it encourages a re-evaluation of their chances of contracting HIV and potentially the discontinuation of PrEP. The ambivalences we observed with queer men resonate with those observed by Rubem da Silva-Brandao and Ianni (2024). Similar to what I have termed 'everyday PrEP negotiations', they observe that queer men engage in 'risk rituals' to manage risk and uncertainties, and note how this ritualisation can complicate their engagement with PrEP.

EIGHT

Liberating, yet constraining

The sixth and final paradox covered in this book relates to PrEP being *both* liberating *and* constraining. The preceding chapters have mentioned some of the many benefits associated with PrEP use, including its ability to eliminate the dark cloud of HIV risk, which taints, or has tainted, the sex lives of our participants. This chapter begins by elaborating on this strong and shared sense of PrEP as liberating. However, ideas about the liberating potential of PrEP are challenged by the recognition of linked constraints, which conjure conflictual ambiguities and tensions. The constraints manifest differently from person to person and between the two study contexts. For both queer men in Denmark and young women in Zimbabwe, the treatment regime – having to take a daily pill and attend regular health checks – was talked about as disruptive and as something that introduced new constraints in their day-to-day lives. For queer men in Denmark, additional constraints included feeling addicted to the sexual freedom and lifestyle that (can) come with PrEP, and recognising the difficulties and complexities related to PrEP discontinuation.

Ideas and ways of thinking about PrEP as both liberating and constraining were found to give rise to everyday PrEP negotiations in the form of handling uncomfortable feelings, difficult considerations, and complex revelations. These will be discussed under the following headings:

- Can I imagine a life without PrEP? Held captive by sexual freedom
- What does PrEP require of me practically? Considering the constraints of PrEP treatment
- When should I stop taking PrEP? Realising the complexities of PrEP discontinuation

Can I imagine a life without PrEP? Held captive by sexual freedom

In this section, I elaborate on the sexual liberation and freedom afforded by PrEP. PrEP users in both contexts express having a newly found sexual freedom when on PrEP, removing feelings of fear of HIV, and providing them with a profound sense of control and autonomy over their sexuality. Chapter 6 has already demonstrated the emancipatory and liberating potential of PrEP in helping queer men and young women safeguard their health. While there is no doubt that PrEP is revolutionary for young women on PrEP, the women who participated in our study did not speak about PrEP in existential terms to the same degree as our queer participants. Queer men had a strong shared understanding of PrEP as revolutionary in liberating their sexuality, stating: 'It really is some kind of sexual revolution', '[I'm] finally able to enjoy sex', 'I feel like a superman', 'having a weight lifted off your shoulder', 'finally peace of mind', 'PrEP makes me feel less abnormal, less of a sinner'. Klaus, who is 42 years old and on PrEP, likened the liberating potential of PrEP to 'coming out of the closet', meaning the process of disclosing your sexual identity, which is empowering and supports queer men in living more open and authentic lives: 'The liberation that comes with PrEP is incomparable with anything else. It is a fantastic feeling. Yes. It feels like coming out of the closet again, for a second time, at the age of 40 [laughs]. That's wild'. Representing PrEP as a liberating force akin to coming out of the closet or having the powers of a superhero, testifies to its existential and transformative capacities. To exemplify this, Bo, a queer man with PrEP experience, describes how PrEP has transformed his relationship with himself and his body:

> PrEP has helped me get a better relationship with myself by accepting who I am and what I do. I've spent a lot of time fighting with myself over the habits I have and the things I do. That it was disgusting, wrong, abnormal, and dangerous. It may well be that it is. But for me, it is also pleasure, freedom, and desire. It is part of the relationship with myself and my body, and it's a part of me and my life. PrEP provides a sense of freedom and worry-free living. (Bo, age 21, PrEP experienced)

For Bo and others, PrEP has come to represent a vehicle for legitimising queer sex, helping them deal with ambiguities related to their internalised stigma and homophobia, and queer sex's association with HIV on the one hand, and the pleasure and desire that come with sex on the other. After years of struggling with such ambivalence, PrEP provides a resolution by eliminating HIV from queer sex and signalling the legitimacy of queer sex. PrEP is thus pivotal to the existential foundation of some queer men. While this is nothing less than remarkable, it creates a context for PrEP dependency and for having difficulties imagining a life without this 'superpower'. No queer person wants to return to the closet. No superhero would want to relinquish their superpower. This dependency contributes to a cascade of constraints and related everyday PrEP negotiations, which I will elaborate upon in the remainder of the chapter.

By way of illustrating this dependency on PrEP, Poul describes his ambiguous relationship with PrEP – one that suggests a constraining reliance on the pills for their intended and liberating purpose. For Poul, it is strenuous to take a daily pill, but he cannot see a way around it to achieve the protection and freedom that it affords:

> Taking PrEP makes me addicted to the pill. I do not have withdrawal symptoms, but I must take it for it to work. You could say it's a voluntary addiction. It's nice to have a drink or two. Then they become 10, and then you have an alcohol problem. And for me, addiction is several things. It can be alcoholism, where you can't help it. And it can be medicine that you must take on a regular basis for it to work. It's a bit unnuanced, but that's how I see it. I prefer to go without. The blue PrEP pill troubles my stomach. But it makes it possible for me to have casual sex with random men in random places. Without having to think about HIV. (Poul, age 46, PrEP user)

The ambiguity that Poul describes illustrates how PrEP involves deliberations about dependency, potential side effects, and the perceived trade-off between taking a pill and the freedom to engage in spontaneous sexual encounters without fear of HIV. However, as illustrated by Holic, dependency on daily pills to achieve PrEP's liberating purpose can lead to another type of constraint, namely a felt obligation to have unprotected sex:

> When I'm on PrEP, I'm more daring. I feel like Superman because I cannot catch the one thing that you cannot cure. When I take it, I may tell myself, 'Oh, I haven't had unprotected sex for two months, and I've been, you know, taking it every day, so why not have unprotected sex?' Then I feel almost like an obligation to have unprotected sex. (Holic, age 32, PrEP user)

Holic relishes the liberation afforded by PrEP, but every day when he takes a pill he is reminded of its purpose. Illustrative of his everyday PrEP negotiations, this makes him deliberate on his HIV vulnerability and the need to stay 'at risk' to reap the advantages of PrEP and justify his practice of taking pills daily.

Overwhelmingly dominant ideas about PrEP's liberating powers to transform the existential foundation of queer sex, body and mind, are not without controversy. They can constrain in subtle ways by fostering a sense of captivity, such as being held captive to daily pill-taking or the need to engage in unprotected sex. In the next section, I further elaborate on some of the considerations of daily pill-taking.

What does PrEP require of me practically? Considering the constraints of PrEP treatment

Prior chapters have already alluded to some of the practical work involved with PrEP use and living up to the 'patient' persona, such as having to go to health checks and PrEP refills at health facilities. This section expands on this therapeutic work, but from the perspective of how PrEP treatment introduces new daily practices and negotiation demands that may be considered restrictive and limiting. Some participants spoke from experience; others drew on shared beliefs and understandings. Either way, people interested in or taking PrEP carefully consider these new demands and weigh them against the liberating and protective benefits of PrEP.

In both study contexts, participants spoke in detail about considerations and difficulties related to PrEP controls and adherence. However, there was considerable variability in the perceived difficulty associated with daily pill-taking. Ashley argued that in Zimbabwe 'People find the idea of taking the daily pill impossible.' In contrast, Lasse, after sharing his challenges with the demands of daily pill-taking in Denmark, said, 'It's just a luxury problem.' By referring to adherence demands (the constraints) as a luxury (the liberation), Lasse neatly summarises the dialectics of the paradox covered in this chapter. These statements by Ashley and Lasse also allude to the varying impacts of these perceived or experienced constraints, with queer men not being impacted by the constraints as much as young women in Zimbabwe. Nonetheless, both queer men and young women spoke in detail about how taking a daily pill is arduous and that PrEP users can easily forget to take it. This was highlighted in a focus group discussion among young women eligible for PrEP in Zimbabwe, where Maria raised the concern that people who are mobile may be particularly susceptible to failing to take their pills:

> I think PrEP is good for people who can adhere to it. People who are mobile tend to forget to carry the pills, even though they are supposed to be taken every day. Even if you remember to carry the pills with you, you may begin to think that you are not even infected with HIV, so why should I take pills every day? That becomes a challenge. (Maria, age 18–24, eligible for PrEP)

Maria also raises the issue that the work involved in remembering to take or bring pills may result in deliberations about the worthiness of this work. Queer men in Denmark also spoke about having difficulties remembering, but in the process remarked on how they had adopted new practices to overcome this challenge. Christian and Toke, for instance, talked about how they had introduced new devices (an app or a pillbox) into their daily routine to support their pill-taking:

> I installed an app on my phone. A medicine app. It comes up with a reminder every day. Otherwise, I forget and know that I have taken the pill. It also ensures that I don't take two pills in one day. So, I think it works well with an app like that. (Christian, age 26, PrEP user)

> Sometimes I was unsure whether I had taken the pill or not. The solution was to buy a pillbox so I could see whether I had taken it. It was a bit difficult to get used to taking a pill every single day, as I don't take any other

medication at all. But now I've thrown in some vitamin pills and some fish oil, which I would not otherwise take because I wouldn't remember. In that way, it has been fine. (Toke, age 27, PrEP user)

What makes daily pill-taking a 'luxury problem' for Toke and Christian is not only that they have access to devices that can help them, but that they can take PrEP every day without fearing repercussions. While daily pill-taking can be a relatively problem-free activity for queer men once they have negotiated the new practice into their daily routine, the regular controls were talked about as more constraining. In Chapter 3 I discussed the opportunity costs associated with time spent going to the hospital during working hours for a routine PrEP control. Negotiating time out of work for PrEP control was noted to be difficult and challenging by several of our participants. Not because they would be denied the time to go, but because it often involved some form of decision-making regarding whether or not to disclose their PrEP use to (some) colleagues. Mike describes his deliberations and the ambivalence he experiences in disclosing his PrEP use to colleagues:

> I actually told a colleague about my PrEP use because I had been to the hospital to have blood tests done, and arrived late to work. To explain myself, I told her that I had been to the hospital, for which she said: 'Well, what ... why are you at the hospital?' So I said, 'Well, I just had a blood test because I've started this medication.' And then she asked, you know, if there was something wrong or ... And I thought: Okay, should I explain this or just say, 'No, nothing is wrong'? And I thought: Oh well, I'll just be completely open and talk about it. I think that has just become my thing to be open and ... what should I say, like, I want to educate other people about PrEP, even those who are not gay, and what HIV means

for gay people in other parts of the world, and what it means for my life and my love life. [...] I think that it has become easier to talk about, so I don't experience any social barriers. (Mike, age 32, PrEP user)

Mike and other queer men may not experience huge hurdles and constraints in telling their sexual partners about their PrEP use, but as a sexual minority, and because of the controversy attached to PrEP, they still need to negotiate whom to disclose their PrEP use to. Many are forced into this negotiation due to PrEP controls taking place during working hours. However, for Mike and two of our other queer participants, this pushed them into instigating important conversations about HIV and the rights of queer people.

The issue of disclosure and whether to keep PrEP use a secret consumed the thoughts of many of the young women participating in our study. As described in the previous chapter, young women described perceived social risks to their PrEP use, if discovered. It was precisely this need to keep PrEP use hidden and secret that was said to necessitate significant levels of deception. This was not only talked about as demanding and exhausting, but also as something that added restriction and constraint to their relationships. The women expressed various and opposing ideas with regards to how demanding this secrecy work was for them. Some, like 22-year-old Elsa, who is eligible for PrEP, believe that keeping PrEP use hidden is possible and a strength of PrEP: 'PrEP is good because you can access it and start taking it without your husband's knowledge, thereby preventing yourself from getting infected with HIV.' However, and as also alluded to in the previous chapter, the task of keeping PrEP use hidden was described by many as insurmountable, as exemplified by Patience and Monica in a focus group discussion:

> They [PrEP pills] are scary to take at home and maybe when you want to take it ... I mean those tablets make

noise ... so you may be heard by your parents, and they would want to know what is going on. (Patience, age 18–24, eligible for PrEP)

When I want to take the pills at home it becomes a challenge because my husband will always be at home. And where to access PrEP in terms of the clinic is another challenge because maybe the nurses won't be secretive and confidential to the extent that when I get home others at home would be knowing already that I went to the local clinic to access PrEP. So, these are some of the challenges that may even lead to divorce. (Monica, age 18–24, eligible for PrEP)

Easy or not, the common belief that young women need to deceive and keep their pill-taking secret also extends into control and PrEP refill visits. One participant said that some young women would have to lie to their husbands to get permission to go to a health centre: 'They would say they want to get a blood test for malaria from the health worker, but then get PrEP there.'

Young women on PrEP reproduced the shared belief and understanding that women need to keep pill-taking secret. They did so by describing how their success and ability to be on PrEP are down to either being able to keep their PrEP use secret or their ability to disclose PrEP use to the people they live with, as exemplified by Esther, who is 22 years old and on PrEP: 'What differentiates me is that after I told the people that I was living with, I was able to take my medication freely without hiding.'

Knowing that medication adherence is pivotal to reaping the protective and liberating benefits of oral PrEP, people either on or contemplating PrEP also consider – as part of their everyday PrEP negotiations – the demands of the daily therapeutic practice of taking pills. For queer men, this was often limited to introducing new devices and practices to support medication adherence, and was not talked about among our participants as a particularly noteworthy constraint on their life. For many young women in Zimbabwe, however, the practical work of taking pills as prescribed, along with storing and handling them and obtaining refills, was considered highly demanding. The women focused on their need to keep their PrEP use hidden and secret, a task that was often perceived as simply too great and constraining for many of the participating women, who worried about the risks of being discovered (see previous chapter).

When should I stop taking PrEP? Realising the complexities of PrEP discontinuation

The ease with which queer men in Denmark or young women in Zimbabwe can stop using PrEP arguably reflects the different demands and constraints imposed by daily pill-taking. Perhaps given the constraints and difficulties affecting young women's access to and use of PrEP, none of them spoke about difficulties with discontinuing PrEP: on the contrary, they felt it was easy. Young women on PrEP appeared to continually evaluate their need for PrEP and were able to decide to discontinue it if they no longer considered themselves vulnerable to HIV, as described by 25-year-old Kimberley, who has experience with PrEP: 'The pills were available, but I saw myself as not at risk of contracting HIV and decided to stop.' However, the reverse was true for queer men, reflecting the power of the liberating effects of PrEP, the hurdles they faced to be deemed eligible, and the relative ease with which they could take PrEP. Thirty-two-year-old Holic is, like Kimberly, beginning to question his vulnerability to HIV, and he has unofficially discontinued PrEP for various short periods. However, as it took him nearly a year to get onto PrEP, or to 'hop on the PrEP train', as he puts it, he is worried about the consequences of officially getting off it:

> I'm afraid it will be difficult to jump back on that train. You know, 'Can I pause it? You don't have to give me

pills now, but I'll call you when I am ready to get back on PrEP again.' So, I don't know what the best strategy is. I would like to get off it, but they made it so difficult the first time around to hop on that train. (Holic, age 32, PrEP user)

Nonetheless, for many of our queer participants, PrEP has become such an existential part of their lives that discontinuing it is beginning to seem inconceivable, but something they questioned through everyday PrEP negotiations, as exemplified by Christian, who captured his pondering through photography (see Figure 8.1):

I want to share this picture to discuss some of my thoughts on how long I should take PrEP. When I started taking PrEP, I thought it would probably just be for a short period while I was single and dating. The idea was that I would stop taking PrEP once I found love and a partner, but after about two years I am still single. I therefore sometimes consider how much sex I have, whether I should have sex with or without a condom, and whether I should continue or stop taking PrEP. (Christian, age 26, PrEP user)

Christian captures a common idea among our queer participants, namely that they will discontinue PrEP when entering a relationship. However, he also alludes to deliberations related to how PrEP, and the sexual liberation that comes with it, may restrain him from entering a relationship. This keeps him on PrEP but also spurs deliberations and negotiations about the need to discontinue PrEP. Mikkel and Lasse also started using PrEP thinking that they would stop when they found love, or as Mikkel put it: 'I will stop when I meet a man and we are not in an open relationship.' Further, Lasse goes on to share that he has observed a norm change within his friendship groups, with more of them living in open relationships and taking advantage

Figure 8.1: 'How long should I take PrEP for?'

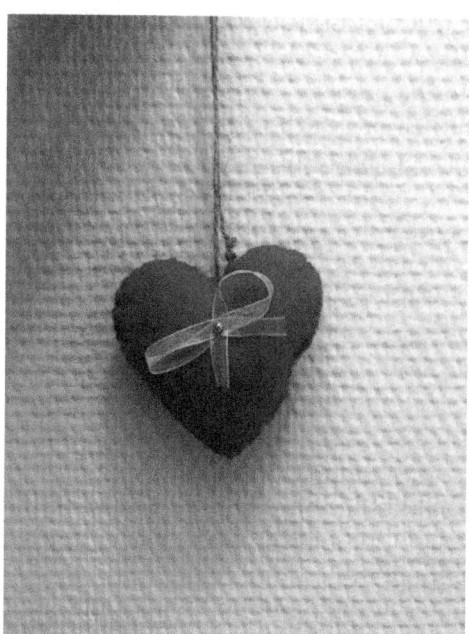

of the sexual freedoms that PrEP enables. This makes Lasse question and feel unsure about the end date of his PrEP use:

> I have two friends who are together in an open relationship and taking PrEP. And I feel that more and more people are in open relationships. So, my idea of finding a partner and stopping PrEP may not hold if my partner and I agree to have an open relationship. But is this something people only do for a period of time, or is it something that most people do for a long time? The end date for when I stop taking PrEP is therefore not easy to predict. I lack information about how long it is recommended to take PrEP and whether it can have any long-term effects. (Lasse, age 25, PrEP user)

This uncertainty and the inconceivability of a so-called end date, while reflecting the liberating powers of PrEP, also spurred Lasse to ask for professional advice on PrEP's long-term use, referring to the possible long-term effects (also discussed in the previous chapter). Christian also talked about the need for information and recommendations about when to stop using PrEP.

In Chapter 5, I referred to PrEP's capacity to create social divisions within the queer community: those on and those not on PrEP, as well as those on PrEP using condoms and those on PrEP not using condoms. These dynamics may carry over into their loving relationships as their openness to having sex with others outside the relationship and (dis)continued PrEP use are negotiated between partners. Feng, for instance, provides details of a conversation he has had with his new partner, who would like Feng to demonstrate his commitment to their monogamous relationship by asking him to stop taking PrEP:

> Yeah, and he was actually encouraging me not to be on PrEP because he wanted us to be monogamous. I said, well, I've been taking PrEP for two years now, and it's become a habit. That doesn't mean I'm just going out to have random sex. I enjoy taking it. I enjoy having this protection. It gives me a sense of security. But he does have a point, I think. Guys taking PrEP every day feel invincible [laughs], and they allow themselves to have random sex. (Feng, age 35, PrEP user)

Feng expresses not only the tension and everyday PrEP negotiations between him and his partner, but also the ambiguity. For Feng, routine PrEP use coexists with the assertion that PrEP does not have to imply engaging in 'random sex', but rather is about feeling protected and secure, *and* recognising how PrEP may in fact result in 'random sex'. Feng captures the dialectics of being both liberated by PrEP through its protection, security, and 'invincibility', and constrained through an almost addiction-like reluctance to discontinue PrEP, which may or may not affect his future relationships.

For queer men in Denmark, the liberating influence of PrEP is potent, so much so that it complicates their journey to get off it. The inconceivability of discontinuing PrEP is not only a constraint in and of itself; it can lead to a cascade of new challenges and everyday negotiations as PrEP enters and comes to reshape queer relationships.

Conclusion

This chapter has outlined how PrEP can offer a sense of liberation and freedom while simultaneously creating dependencies or constraints in new and various ways. This chapter, more than any other, explores how PrEP can influence and transform identities, relationships, and sexual practices, highlighting the powerful role it plays in shaping these aspects of people's lives. PrEP is thus not merely a pill but a sociocultural phenomenon with meanings and consequences for how people live their lives. In other words, PrEP works *on* people. PrEP's capacity to liberate was vividly depicted in the testimonies of our queer male participants, most of whom have experience with PrEP and navigate social networks in which PrEP is increasingly used. From their accounts, it is clear that PrEP has entered the hearts and minds of many queer networks in Denmark and is associated with a profound sense of autonomy, sexual freedom, and self-acceptance. As also argued by Punchihewa et al. (2024) based on research with queer men in New Zealand, PrEP cannot be reduced to only being about the prevention of HIV. The sex that PrEP enables has an intrinsic value, both in terms of pleasure and freedom, and for the expression of identity. While our young female participants fully recognised the liberating potential of PrEP, this was primarily from the perspective of not having to worry about HIV and being able to take control over their lives. For Zimbabwean heterosexual women, PrEP does not therefore appear to be *as* consequential or existential as it is for queer men in Denmark. However positive this liberation may be, it is not without its contradictions.

For queer men in Denmark, and in many other parts of the Global North, PrEP can become so entrenched in their lives and carry such significant meaning that they begin to feel a sense of dependency on it, akin to addiction. This instigates deliberation and a realisation of how PrEP not only gives them control over the risks of having condomless anal sex, but also controls their lives. Aside from the sense of dependency itself, this includes not being able to listen to their body reacting negatively to pill-taking, or staying in the 'fast lane' by having numerous sexual encounters because of a sense of the perverse obligation to 'stay at risk'. PrEP's influence on their lives also emerged when contemplating PrEP discontinuation. There was a collective understanding that PrEP would be naturally discontinued when entering a serious relationship. However, upon further reflection, and because of PrEP's impact above and beyond HIV prevention, this was described as difficult and likely to result in a discussion with their future partner about their continued PrEP use. Given the different and divisive ways of thinking about PrEP – including within the queer community, as discussed in Chapter 5 – their perspectives on partner reactions gave rise to ambiguity and uncertainty. It also sparked reflection on how this need to negotiate continued PrEP use may determine the nature of the queer men's future relationships, including their openness to having sex with other men outside of their relationships.

Another constraint relates to the arduous and practical work of daily pill-taking. While queer men in Denmark did mention pill-taking as demanding, they were able to introduce tools and practices that would ease this work, making it less of a constraint. Young women in Zimbabwe, on the other hand, gave countless examples of how difficult and challenging it is for them to take a daily PrEP pill. As a result of a perceived widespread lack of social acceptance of PrEP among parents and partners, there was a shared understanding that many young women would need to keep their pill-taking secret and hidden from their partners. For the young women, having to lie to and deceive their partners was described as difficult and something that came with great social risks (as discussed in the previous chapter). While some of the young women on PrEP had disclosed their PrEP use to partners or even took up PrEP *with* their partners, the shared idea that most male partners would disapprove of their female partners' PrEP use was all-consuming for young women interested in PrEP, necessitating PrEP negotiations. Irrespective of whether they are considering or already taking PrEP secretly, this idea affects how they view their partner and their relationship. Young women in Zimbabwe thus also give detail to a shared understanding of PrEP potentially impacting romantic relationships in new and unforeseen ways.

NINE

PrEP paradoxes: problematic, yet productive

This concluding chapter summarises and discusses my analysis, starting with headline findings that cut across both study contexts. This takes me to a discussion of the origins of the PrEP paradoxes, key differences between the two study contexts, and what this means for efforts looking to make PrEP work for more people.

I end the chapter by reflecting on lessons to be learnt for preventive medicine more broadly. This includes an emphasis on the value of some of the language and concepts introduced in this book in expanding and advancing our understanding of the 'problematic, yet productive' nature of paradoxes in making preventive medicine in general work for more people.

Headline findings

How do queer men in Denmark and young straight women in Zimbabwe encounter, respond to, and negotiate PrEP use? This was the overarching question guiding the generation of data for the two case studies presented in this book. As we analysed the data, we quickly learnt that both population groups, despite their many differences, had something in common: they *encountered* opposing ideas and ways of thinking about PrEP. I therefore constructed six paradoxical statements (the headings of Chapters 3–8) that sought to capture the essence of these encounters, while also suggesting that our study participants dialectically struggle with the following:

- PrEP is free to them (in both contexts), yet associated with costs.
- They are eligible for PrEP, yet have their eligibility challenged.
- They take responsibility for their sexual health, yet are confronted with ideas about engaging in irresponsible sexual behaviour (only applicable for queer men in Denmark).
- They are healthy, yet required to adopt a 'patient' persona.
- PrEP keeps them safe from contracting HIV, yet is associated with other risks and harm.
- PrEP offers a strong sense of sexual freedom and liberation, yet is also associated with many new constraints.

These PrEP paradoxes led to contentions, uncertainties, dilemmas, and ambiguities that had to be *responded* to and *negotiated* in each person's everyday context. I thus framed and structured the book according to what I term 'everyday PrEP negotiations' (see Box 1.1, Chapter 1). These everyday PrEP negotiations took different forms and involved:

- sense-making;
- realising, balancing, or weighing up difficult choices and considerations;
- instigating critical thinking;
- dealing with feelings of fear, concern, entrapment, and shame;
- navigating or reconciling opposing ideas;
- questioning or rethinking PrEP as a pill that affects their social and sexual lives;
- 'othering' and following social identity processes.

While I have alluded to some of the practical work involved with oral PrEP, such as daily pill-taking or difficulties in finding transport to health facilities – topics that have been extensively covered in the 'barriers to PrEP' literature – the listed everyday PrEP negotiations reveal the need for a very different type of work, namely 'mental work'. This hitherto hidden form of work complicates and adds to the burden of treatment. A key contribution of this book is that it recognises and makes visible the mental work involved with PrEP and demonstrates how such labour is amplified by PrEP paradoxes, determining people's different abilities to engage with PrEP. However, what the book also shows is that PrEP paradoxes are socially constructed, sometimes intentionally through the negotiations that take place in everyday life among peers, family, and healthcare providers. This suggests that there can be value in PrEP paradoxes and that they are part of the journey and process of developing the form of sense-making that establishes PrEP as a possible and desirable thing to incorporate into their lives. I will now expand on these headline findings and, in the process, tease out differences between the two study contexts. I start with a discussion of how PrEP paradoxes come to be.

Social representations, the moralising of sexuality, and the construction of PrEP paradoxes

The many paradoxical ideas and ways of thinking that our participants encountered did not emerge out of thin air, nor indeed did they merely manifest in their heads. On the contrary, they reflect an assemblage of social representations, meaning the shared beliefs, ideas, values, and practices that circulate in their communities, and in turn frame how our participants understand and talk about PrEP. Many of these representations cast light on how societies moralise sexuality. I will give some examples.

Young women in Zimbabwe, for instance, had to navigate strong social representations about what it means to be a 'good girl'. Ideas and ways of thinking about how to be and act like a good girl – rooted in a patriarchal public gender order that discourages extra- and premarital sex among adolescent girls and young women – stand in stark contrast to PrEP, which perversely was represented as an HIV prevention method for sex workers or women with so-called loose morals. Aside from signalling promiscuity or infidelity, it was also said to signal women's lack of trust in their male partners. Against this background there were social representations about the social risks and negative reactions of parents, partners, and PrEP service providers if they discovered the young women's PrEP use. The representation of the low social acceptability of PrEP along with fear of social risks remained a strong shared meaning, and, arguably, a critical determinant of PrEP uptake and utilisation. Yet at the same time peers, public campaigns, and HIV prevention service providers were actively constructing positive social representations about PrEP as free, effective, and capable of helping women control their vulnerability to HIV. The young women participating in our study had encountered these representations also, and described them in their expressions of support for and interest in using PrEP. Herein lies the construction of PrEP paradoxes and an example of some of the battles of ideas that young women in Zimbabwe must negotiate in their everyday lives.

Queer men in Denmark also had to navigate social representations centred around a prevailing, taken-for-granted understanding of moral and sexual conduct. Social representations of 'good' or 'normal' sexual conduct not only contribute to internalised homophobia and PrEP-related stigma within the queer community, but also frame public debates about PrEP and queer sexuality in the media. As such, our queer participants encountered a variety of value-driven social representations about who a PrEP user is, both within and outside the queer community. Similar to what has been identified in the USA (Spieldenner, 2016) and in the British press (Jaspal and Nerlich, 2017), they include but are not limited to being: promiscuous and a so-called Truvada whore; a person looking for a ticket to condomless anal sex; and an expense to society for their 'risky' sexual behaviour and for contributing to increases in sexually transmitted infections. While such representations of a PrEP user obstruct access to PrEP for some queer men, for others they ignite counter-ideas. The queer men participating in this study were found to develop new shared meanings about PrEP and the centralised organisation of PrEP services in Denmark, including the policy framework in place to determine PrEP eligibility. Strict eligibility controls and the focus on *past* HIV risk behaviour were found to reproduce representations of PrEP as an expensive drug whose use should be limited and only made available to queer men who demonstrably need to treat their sexuality and infectious disease risk. Yet at the same time, the queer community had constructed, through social interactions, a new shared language and common understandings of PrEP as revolutionary in liberating their sexuality: representations of PrEP as health-, life-, and sexuality-promoting thus also infused our accounts from queer men. Again, herein lies the construction of PrEP paradoxes and the need for queer men's everyday PrEP negotiations.

The examples I have given illustrate how society's moralising of sexuality both forms and maintains assemblages of social representations of what constitutes 'good' and 'moral' sexual conduct. In Zimbabwe, these strongly intersect with gender orders and indicate that the moral codes that apply respectively to men and women are different. In Denmark, on the other hand, these representations intersect with sexual identity and how the social welfare state governs and controls PrEP. While both groups face challenges to PrEP uptake and utilisation, they are hardly comparable. The challenges faced by many young women in Zimbabwe are often unsurmountable. Obviously, many different individual and socio-cultural factors play into this, including relationship status, patriarchy, poverty, and the patriarchal culture of which they form a part. However, the dominance and stability of moralising social representations about PrEP and sexuality in Zimbabwe appear to play a central role in obstructing young women's uptake and utilisation of PrEP. In Denmark, for many queer men – who have more independence, form part of a liberal society, and have a history of challenging heteronormativity – moralising social representations appear to merely complicate, rather than inhibit, PrEP use. For, while moralising social representations about PrEP and sexuality do also flourish in Denmark and prevent some queer men and transpersons from accessing PrEP, they are more openly contested and evolving, and do not appear to be as consequential, at least for our study participants. In this context, and with a supportive social network, it is easier for queer men to counter and resist harmful representations by themselves transforming the values or beliefs that guide their interpretations, meaning-making, and actions with regards to PrEP.

By comparing the different opposing ideas and ways of thinking that young straight women in Zimbabwe and queer men in Denmark encounter about PrEP, the evolving nature of social representations and their dynamic influence on PrEP paradoxes become clear. Slow but shifting societal attitudes (for example, with regards to gender orders or sexual orientations), the media and public debates, health communication and campaigns, social interactions and debates among groups of individuals – all these offer counter-ideas and new ways of thinking. They contribute to PrEP paradoxes and periods of liminality in which contention, uncertainty, dilemmas, and ambiguity profoundly shape motivation and action to take up PrEP, or indeed shape experiences of using PrEP and necessitate everyday PrEP negotiation – a form of mental work. However, it is through this mental work that PrEP users may learn or accept that opposing ideas can coexist or further form and reproduce ideas and ways of thinking that help them interpret and make sense of PrEP in ways that support their uptake and utilisation of it. This offers a segue into a discussion of how to make PrEP work for more people.

Making PrEP 'work for' more people: the roles of social networks

In the Introduction and building on the work of Auerbach and Hoppe (2015), I made the case for an approach to PrEP delivery that seeks to understand and respond to what it takes to get PrEP to work for more people. My focus on the *work involved* with PrEP and how PrEP *works on* people has identified PrEP as an inherently social practice that, in the context of users' everyday and social lives, involves intense mental work and can affect how they live their lives. This insight offers important clues for making PrEP work for more people. While the findings presented in this book point to many different avenues of socio-behavioural intervention, social networks appear to play an integral role in making PrEP work for people. Inspired by the work of Campbell et al. (2013) I now outline five social psychological processes that I noted are facilitated and supported by social networks in the form of sense-making, and that establish PrEP as something that works for them as individuals and as a collective.

First, social networks create spaces for *engaging in critical dialogue and thinking about PrEP*. People interested in or using PrEP talk to each other. They exchange opportunities and challenges to access and openly discuss how PrEP could be delivered differently. Queer men, for instance, as part of their individual and collective sense-making process, engaged in critical dialogue about the rigidity and centralisation of PrEP services in Denmark. Sharing experiences and perspectives also helps people feel more confident to engage in dialogue about sensitive or controversial topics, such as when young women in Zimbabwe talked about their sexuality and the risks of using PrEP, or when queer men in Denmark talked about PrEP (ir)responsibilities or the practice of lying to healthcare providers. By sharing experiences and ways of thinking about what makes PrEP an (im)possible or (un)desirable thing to incorporate into their lives, certain values, ideas, or practices gain traction and (il)legitimacy, deepening people's sense-making and the meanings they ascribe to PrEP.

Second, critical dialogue with peers creates a context for *co-constructing new norms, values, and beliefs about PrEP*, which make PrEP workable for them. Queer men in Denmark, for example, reformulated eligibility away from a focus on past risk to future risk-taking. They also made it an acceptable norm to tell little white lies to circumvent ineligibility from a PrEP service provider perspective. They were also able to reframe negative expressions such as 'slut-shaming' into something positive. However, social networks can also reproduce unhelpful beliefs, as was noted among our young female participants in Zimbabwe. They inadvertently reproduced ideas about the negative implications of PrEP use. While there is no doubt that some young women face real risks because of the low social acceptability of PrEP, particularly from their partners, growing evidence suggests that parents are often more supportive of their adolescent children taking PrEP than adolescents give them credit for (Giovenco et al., 2023; Skovdal et al., 2023). Despite such evidence, and the fact that our recent work in Zimbabwe notes changes in socio-cultural norms and greater lenience towards young women's sexuality (Gregson et al., 2024), the resilience of gender norms as they are reproduced through re-presentation of the social risks of PrEP call for community interventions that involve parents, partners, and healthcare providers as allies in the delivery of PrEP. A similar call has been made by Katz et al. (2023) based on research with young women in Kenya and South Africa.

Third, social networks also provide context for *constructing positive social identities around PrEP use* and the sexual capital that comes with it. Young female PrEP users in Zimbabwe were found to construct a positive social identity as someone who is able to limit their chances of contracting HIV and does not succumb to PrEP-related stigma. Queer men in

Denmark were found to 'other' non-PrEP users and developed favourable biases as a way of responding to the dialectics of (ir)responsibility. In this process, however, queer men may inadvertently stigmatise non-PrEP users and create divisions within the queer community – dynamics that Haire et al. (2021) have also noted among queer men in Australia.

Fourth, I also found that social networks offer important context for *promoting solidarity and social support*. Young female PrEP users in Zimbabwe, as a result of the gendered challenges they face in taking up and using PrEP, created a form of sisterhood characterised by social support, such as going for PrEP pill refills together. Queer men, on the other hand, reflected on the fact that they form part of a larger community and that their access to PrEP is a result of a history of fighting for their rights. Many felt an obligation to safeguard these rights and saw it as their duty to educate others about PrEP and to break down taboos. Burgeoning research with different PrEP target groups is highlighting the important role of social support structures in facilitating engagement with PrEP (Wood et al., 2020; Felsher et al., 2021; Zapata et al., 2022), and research from Australia has also found queer men to be actively engaged in the promotion of PrEP in their social circles (Haire et al., 2021).

Last, social networks provide context for *meaning-making about PrEP's capacity to win hearts and minds*. In both study contexts, participants co-constructed narratives about how PrEP is liberating them from past struggles, evoking both emotive and logical appeals. For queer men in Denmark, the logical appeal of reducing vulnerability to HIV for themselves and others was important, but more so was the emotive appeal that came with the removal of the black cloud and fear that had for decades tainted both their sexuality and the ensuing sexual liberation. For young women in Zimbabwe, being able to control their vulnerability to HIV and not rely on their partners' condom use was talked about as appealing. However, the many social challenges they face in taking up and using PrEP complicate its emotive appeal.

The five social psychological processes outlined here both form part of and, with time, help attenuate the struggles and mental work involved with everyday PrEP negotiations. Following Campbell et al.'s (2007) conceptualisation of the 'AIDS-competent community', this suggests that social networks that are able to facilitate such social psychological processes can be characterised as 'PrEP-competent social networks'. A PrEP-competent social network can thus be defined as a social network that i) enables PrEP users to engage in critical dialogue and thinking; ii) co-constructs new social norms, values, and beliefs and social identities; iii) forms positive social identities around PrEP use; iv) promotes solidarity and social support; and v) gives meaning to PrEP's capacity to capture hearts and minds.

Because oral PrEP, the ways in which it is delivered via hospitals or sexual health clinics, and the different ways of thinking that exist 'out there' do not always resonate with the lived realities of PrEP users, these social psychological processes – and PrEP-competent social networks – appear to be central to making PrEP work for people. However, crucially, they appear to involve constructing and engaging with new ideas and ways of thinking. In other words, PrEP paradoxes are part and parcel of the process of making PrEP work for people. This brings me to the final paradox of the book, namely that PrEP paradoxes are problematic, yet also productive.

PrEP paradoxes: problematic, yet productive

There are three main reasons why PrEP paradoxes are problematic. First, PrEP paradoxes are indicative of the resilience and dominance of unhelpful ideas and ways of thinking that establish PrEP as an impossible and undesirable thing to incorporate into some people's lives. Second, PrEP paradoxes contribute to contention, uncertainty, dilemmas, and ambiguity, which demand substantial mental work through everyday PrEP negotiations. This may not only lead to paralysis, a form of 'stuckness' and inaction around PrEP use, as seen among many of our young female participants from Zimbabwe, but also contribute to inequities in uptake and use depending on the PrEP competence of their respective social networks (as mentioned earlier). Third, PrEP paradoxes are problematic because of their reminiscence or amplification of the struggles of sexual minorities and women in the Global South. Although it would be preferable if people vulnerable to HIV could access PrEP without having to consider obstructive ideas and ways of thinking, this is still not the case for most people. While this is highly problematic and goes some way to explaining why PrEP does not work for many people, it is not the whole story.

PrEP paradoxes can also play a productive role, and I would like to submit two reasons for this. First, PrEP paradoxes appear to be part of a process and are illustrative of resistance to ways of thinking that are counterproductive. As a collective, PrEP users deliberately introduce new and alternative ideas and ways of thinking that make PrEP work for them. With time and through everyday PrEP negotiations, particularly in the context of PrEP-competent social networks, these ideas gain greater legitimacy, which makes the uncertainties and dilemmas more manageable, and makes PrEP work for more users. However, although people on PrEP may have come to a resolution, their awareness of opposing ideas will remain (cognitive polyphasia), affecting their experiences and whether or not they continue to take PrEP. This was seen among many of our queer male participants in Denmark. Second, PrEP paradoxes and ensuing everyday PrEP negotiations may energise PrEP users to stay engaged, as they trigger thought and reflection, which, according to Marková (1987), is critical to deepening their knowledge and commitment to a cause – in this case, taking PrEP.

What does this mean for PrEP service delivery and public health practice? First, PrEP paradoxes and the visibility of the mental work required of PrEP users *have to* inform the delivery of PrEP services. This involves developing both services that take heed of the findings presented in this book and person-centred care practices that pay attention to how PrEP paradoxes manifest and shape PrEP uptake and utilisation. For the former, I have noted many contentions that could be easily responded to. For Denmark, this includes increasing opening hours and decentralising PrEP services, as well as expanding eligibility criteria to include those with the future intention of taking risks. For Zimbabwe, it may include eliminating costs associated with accessing PrEP, developing youth-friendly services, and avoiding delivering PrEP through the same clinics that deliver treatment for HIV. It may also include interventions to rectify misperceptions, albeit only if research indicates that this is the case.

Second, the need for PrEP-competent social networks calls for what Kippax and Stephenson (2012) have referred to as a 'social public health' response. Such a response would recognise the agency of a collective, and support community engagement efforts aimed at strengthening the PrEP competence of social networks, making PrEP 'work for' more people.

Third, efforts looking to expand PrEP uptake and utilisation must include social marketing and health campaigns that endorse and promote ideas and ways of thinking about PrEP that resonate with PrEP user target groups, and simultaneously challenge counterproductive ideas and ways of thinking that circulate in the public sphere.

Paradoxes and everyday disease prevention negotiations

Much preventive medicine relates to diseases that may rather simplistically be considered lifestyle-related, such as HIV (related to sexual behaviour), lung cancer (linked to smoking), and obesity and cardiometabolic diseases (linked to diet and physical activity patterns). There is only a short step from attaching moral responsibility for so-called unhealthy and lifestyle-related behaviours to medication stigma. As a result, many disease prevention medications are steeped in controversy. Users of such medications may encounter attitudes and ways of thinking that further complicate and heighten the need for everyday disease prevention negotiations. Looking at weight loss medication, Haggerty et al. (2023: p 3240) find that the language used on X (Twitter, as was) to communicate about weight loss medication is stigmatising approximately half the time. They note that people assign blame and responsibility to users of weight loss medications, stereotyping them as lazy and taking the 'easy way out'. Societal costs and the burden on healthcare systems were also observed to be publicly communicated. People struggling with overweight inevitably encounter such moralising ideas and ways of thinking. This may give rise to difficult questions and dilemmas concerning their eligibility and deservedness, the costs involved, as well as the effortfulness and sustainability of their weight loss (Oswald, 2024).

Although this book has focused on PrEP for the prevention of HIV, I would argue that paradoxes form the context of much preventive medicine and that key takeaways from this book thus also apply to other areas of pharmaceutical prevention. Where stigma and moralising public debates are part of the social landscape, or where preventive medication introduces interferences into daily life, users will inevitably encounter conflicting ideas and ways of thinking. As a result, they may dialectically experience contention, uncertainty, dilemmas, or ambiguity. To make preventive medication work for them, individuals will need to engage in 'everyday disease prevention negotiations' – both internally, through subtle mental activities, and externally, with peers, family, and healthcare providers who can help them reflect on, challenge, or reinforce certain ideas, practices, or norms related to the medication.

As I have shown, pharmaceutical prevention involves much more than simply taking a pill. It requires significant mental work in the form of everyday disease prevention negotiations, which, paradoxically can be both problematic and productive.

However, the burden of this mental work can be eased by supportive social networks. This, as well as the social nature of how ideas and ways of thinking take root within a particular group or society, suggests that individuals have different prerequisites for making preventive medicine *work for* them, and highlights the need for social public health interventions.

Notes

one
[1] Video capturing the optimism of AIDS 2012 conference: https://youtu.be/jeaUP_vuOLE
[2] For an overview of PrEP products under development: https://www.prepwatch.org/research-pipeline
[3] https://vimeo.com/323748000

References

Attride-Stirling, J. (2001) 'Thematic networks: An analytic tool for qualitative research', *Qualitative Research*, 1: 385–405.

Auerbach, J.D. and Hoppe, T.A. (2015) 'Beyond "getting drugs into bodies": Social science perspectives on pre-exposure prophylaxis for HIV', *Journal of the International AIDS Society*, 18: 19983.

Auvert, B., Taljaard, D., Lagarde, E., Sobngwi-Tambekou, J., Sitta, R., and Puren, A. (2005) 'Randomized, controlled intervention trial of male circumcision for reduction of HIV infection risk: The ANRS 1265 Trial', *PLoS Medicine*, 2(11): e298. doi: 10.1371/journal.pmed.0020298.

Bagge-Petersen, C.M. (2023) 'Living ambivalently with chronic illness', *Medical Anthropology*, 42: 191–205.

Bagge-Petersen, C.M., Skovdal, M., and Langstrup, H. (2020) 'The socio-material self-care practices of children living with hemophilia or juvenile idiopathic arthritis in Denmark', *Social Science & Medicine*, 255: 113022.

Bernays, S., Bourne, A., Kippax, S., Aggleton, P., and Parker, R. (2021) 'Remaking HIV prevention: The promise of TasP, U=U and PrEP', in S. Bernays, A. Bourne, S. Kippax, P. Aggleton, and R. Parker (eds), *Remaking HIV Prevention in the 21st Century: The Promise of TasP, U=U and PrEP*, Cham: Springer International Publishing, pp 1–18.

Billig, M. (1996) *Arguing and Thinking: A Rhetorical Approach to Social Psychology*, Cambridge: Cambridge University Press.

Birk, H., Vrangbæk, K., Rudkjøbing, A., Krasnik, A., Eriksen, A., Richardson, E., et al. (2024) 'Denmark: Health system review', *Health Systems in Transition*, 26: i–152.

Brisson, J. and Nguyen, V.-K. (2017) 'Science, technology, power and sex: PrEP and HIV-positive gay men in Paris', *Culture, Health & Sexuality*, 19: 1066–77.

BT (2016) 'Økonom: Dyr hiv-behandling overskrider statens ansvar', 13 May 2016, Available from: www.bt.dk/danmark/oekonom-dyr-hiv-behandling-overskrider-statens-ansvar-0 [Accessed 28 November 2024].

Cambiano, V., Miners, A., Dunn, D., McCormack, S., Ong, K.J., Gill, O.N., et al. (2018) 'Cost-effectiveness of pre-exposure prophylaxis for HIV prevention in men who have sex with men in the UK: A modelling study and health economic evaluation', *The Lancet Infectious Diseases*, 18: 85–94.

Campbell, C., Nair, Y., and Maimane, S. (2007) 'Building contexts that support effective community responses to HIV/AIDS: A South African case study', *American Journal of Community Psychology*, 39: 347–63.

Campbell, C., Scott, K., Nhamo, M., Nyamukapa, C., Madanhire, C., Skovdal, M., et al. (2013) 'Social capital and HIV competent communities: The role of community groups in managing HIV/AIDS in rural Zimbabwe', *AIDS Care*, 25: S114–S122.

Chang, A.Y., Maswera, R., Moorhouse, L.R., Skovdal, M., Nyamukapa, C., and Gregson, S. (2021) 'The determinants and impacts of age-disparate relationships on women in Zimbabwe: A life course perspective', *SSM-Population Health*, 16: 100947.

Chibango, V. and Potgieter, C. (2023) 'Patriarchy, couple counselling and testing in preventing mother-to-child transmission of HIV in Zimbabwe', *HTS Teologiese Studies/Theological Studies*, 79: 7891.

Cluver, L.D., Orkin, M.F., Yakubovich, A.R., and Sherr, L. (2016) 'Combination social protection for reducing HIV-risk behavior amongst adolescents in South Africa', *Journal of Acquired Immune Deficiency Syndromes (1999)*, 72: 96.

REFERENCES

Cohen, M.S., Chen, Y.Q., McCauley, M., Gamble, T., Hosseinipour, M.C., Kumarasamy, N., et al. (2011) 'Prevention of HIV-1 infection with early antiretroviral therapy', *New England Journal of Medicine*, 365: 493–505.

Corbin, J. and Strauss, A. (1985) 'Managing chronic illness at home: Three lines of work', *Qualitative Sociology*, 8: 224–47.

Cornish, F., Gillespie, A., and Zittoun, T. (2013) 'Collaborative analysis of qualitative data', in U. Flick (ed), *The SAGE Handbook of Qualitative Data Analysis*, London: Sage, pp 79–93.

Dean, T. (2015) 'Mediated intimacies: Raw sex, Truvada, and the biopolitics of chemoprophylaxis', *Sexualities*, 18: 224–46.

Defty, J., Wagland, R., and Richardson, A. (2023) 'Understanding the urgent and emergency care navigation work undertaken by people with cancer and their informal caregivers: A conceptually framed scoping review', *Emergency Cancer Care*, 2: 2.

Demetriou, D.Z. (2001) 'Connell's concept of hegemonic masculinity: A critique', *Theory and Society*, 30: 337–61.

Dourado, I., Magno, L., Soares, F., Massa, P., Nunn, A., Dalal, S., et al. (2020) 'Adapting to the COVID-19 pandemic: Continuing HIV prevention services for adolescents through telemonitoring, Brazil', *AIDS and Behavior*, 24: 1994–9.

Durand-Zaleski, I., Mutuon, P., Charreau, I., Tremblay, C., Rojas, D., Pialoux, G., et al. (2018) 'Costs and benefits of on-demand HIV preexposure prophylaxis in MSM', *AIDS*, 32: 95–102.

Ellis, C., Kiesinger, C.E., and Tillmann-Healy, L.M. (1997) 'Interactive interviewing: Talking about emotional experience', in R. Hertz (ed), *Reflexivity and Voice*, London: Sage Publications, pp 119–49.

Engsig, F.N. and Kronborg, G. (2024) 'Forebyggende behandling mod hiv-infektion', *Ugeskr Læger*, 186: V10230672.

Farr, R. (1987) 'Social representations: A French tradition of research', *Journal for the Theory of Social Behaviour*, 17(4): 343–69.

Felsher, M., Dutra, K., Monseur, B., Roth, A.M., Latkin, C., and Falade-Nwulia, O. (2021) 'The influence of PrEP-related stigma and social support on PrEP-use disclosure among women who inject drugs and social network members', *AIDS and Behavior*, 25: 3922–32.

Fidan, A. and Bui, H.N. (2016) 'Intimate partner violence against women in Zimbabwe', *Violence Against Women*, 22: 1075–96.

Flyvbjerg, B. (2006) 'Five misunderstandings about case-study research', *Qualitative Inquiry*, 12: 219–45.

Frescura, L., Godfrey-Faussett, P., Feizzadeh, A.A., El-Sadr, W., Syarif, O., and Ghys, P.D. (2022) 'Achieving the 95 95 95 targets for all: A pathway to ending AIDS', *PLoS One*, 17: e0272405.

Gammeltoft, T.M., Bùi, T.H.D., Vũ, T.K.D., Vũ, Đ.A., Nguyễn, T.Á., and Lê, M.H. (2022) 'Everyday disease diplomacy: An ethnographic study of diabetes self-care in Vietnam', *BMC Public Health*, 22: 1–9.

García-Iglesias, J. (2022) '"PrEP is like an adult using floaties": Meanings and new identities of PrEP among a niche sample of gay men', *Culture, Health & Sexuality*, 24: 153–66.

Giovenco, D., Pettifor, A., Bekker, L.-G., Filiatreau, L.M., Liu, T., Akande, M., et al. (2023) 'Understanding oral prep interest among South African adolescents: The role of perceived parental support and PrEP stigma', *AIDS and Behavior*, 27: 1906–13.

Girometti, N., Delpech, V., McCormack, S., Khawam, J., Nash, S., Ogaz, D., et al. (2021) 'The success of HIV combination prevention: The Dean Street model', *HIV Medicine*, 22: 892–7.

Gourlay, A., Birdthistle, I., Mthiyane, N.T., Orindi, B.O., Muuo, S., Kwaro, D., et al. (2019) 'Awareness and uptake of layered HIV prevention programming for young women: Analysis of population-based surveys in three DREAMS settings in Kenya and South Africa', *BMC Public Health*, 19: 1417.

REFERENCES

Gregson, S., Moorhouse, L., Maswera, R., Dadirai, T., Magoge-Mandizvidza, P., Skovdal, M., et al. (2024) 'Social norms and structural barriers to use of HIV prevention in unmarried and married young women in Manicaland, Zimbabwe: An HIV prevention cascade analysis', Gates Open Research (https://doi.org/10.12688/gatesopenres.15127.1) [Accessed 14 November 2024].

Grulich, A.E., Jin, F., Bavinton, B.R., Yeung, B., Hammoud, M.A., Amin, J., et al. (2021) 'Long-term protection from HIV infection with oral HIV pre-exposure prophylaxis in gay and bisexual men: Findings from the expanded and extended EPIC-NSW prospective implementation study', *The Lancet HIV*, 8: e486–e494.

Haaland, I., Metta, E., and Moen, K. (2023), 'The use of PrEP among men who have sex with men and transgender women as biomedical prevention work: A conceptual framework', *Social Science & Medicine*, 333: 116147.

Haggerty, T., Sedney, C.L., Cowher, A., Holland, D., Davisson, L., and Dekeseredy, P. (2023) 'Twitter and communicating stigma about medications to treat obesity', *Health Communication*, 38: 3238–42.

Haire, B., Murphy, D., Maher, L., Zablotska-Manos, I., Vaccher, S., and Kaldor, J. (2021) 'What does PrEP mean for 'safe sex' norms? A qualitative study', *PLoS One*, 16: e0255731.

Harawa, N.T., Holloway, I.W., Leibowitz, A., Weiss, R., Gildner, J., Landovitz, R.J., et al. (2017) 'Serious concerns regarding a meta-analysis of preexposure prophylaxis use and STI acquisition', *AIDS*, 31: 739–40.

Hawkes, N. (2016) 'NHS England blames possible legal action for decision not to fund HIV prevention pill', *BMJ*, 352: i1708.

Hayes, R.J., Donnell, D., Floyd, S., Mandla, N., Bwalya, J., Sabapathy, K., et al. (2019), 'Effect of universal testing and treatment on HIV incidence—HPTN 071 (PopART)', *New England Journal of Medicine*, 381: 207–18.

Hedrick, A.M. and Carpentier, F.R.D. (2021) 'How current and potential pre-exposure prophylaxis (PrEP) users experience, negotiate and manage stigma: disclosures and backstage processes in online discourse', *Culture, Health & Sexuality*, 23: 1079–93.

Hill, B.J., Anderson, B., and Lock, L. (2021) 'COVID-19 pandemic, pre-exposure prophylaxis (PrEP) care, and HIV/STI testing among patients receiving care in three HIV epidemic priority states', *AIDS and Behavior*, 25: 1361–5.

Iwuji, C.C., Orne-Gliemann, J., Larmarange, J., Balestre, E., Thiebaut, R., Tanser, F., et al. (2018) 'Universal test and treat and the HIV epidemic in rural South Africa: A phase 4, open-label, community cluster randomised trial', *The Lancet HIV*, 5: e116–e125.

Jaspal, R. and Nerlich, B. (2017) 'Polarised press reporting about HIV prevention: Social representations of pre-exposure prophylaxis in the UK press', *Health*, 21: 478–97.

Joffe, H. (2002) 'Social representations and health psychology', *Social Science Information*, 41: 559–80.

Jovchelovitch, S. (2007) *Knowledge in Context: Representations, Community, and Culture*, New York, NY: Routledge.

Jowsey, T., Yen, L., and W, P.M. (2012) 'Time spent on health related activities associated with chronic illness: A scoping literature review', *BMC Public Health*, 12: 1044.

Kambarami, M. (2006) *Femininity, Sexuality and Culture: Patriarchy and Female Subordination in Zimbabwe*, University of Fort Hare, South Africa (http://www.arsrc.org/downloads/uhsss/kmabarami.pdf): Africa Regional Sexuality Resource Centre [Accessed 2 September 2024].

Katz, A.W.K., Roberts, S., Rousseau, E., Khoza, M.N., Mogaka, F., Bukusi, E., et al. (2023) 'Qualitative analysis using social maps to explore young women's experiences with social support of their oral PrEP use in Kenya and South Africa', *Journal of the Association of Nurses in AIDS Care*, 34: 45–57.

Kerzner, M., De, A.K., Yee, R., Keating, R., Djomand, G., Stash, S., et al. (2022) 'Pre-exposure prophylaxis (PrEP) uptake and service delivery adaptations during the first wave of the COVID-19 pandemic in 21 PEPFAR-funded countries', *PLoS One*, 17: e0266280.

REFERENCES

Kippax, S. (2012) 'Effective HIV prevention: the indispensable role of social science', *Journal of the International AIDS Society*, 15(2): 17357.

Kippax, S. and Stephenson, N. (2012) 'Beyond the distinction between biomedical and social dimensions of HIV prevention through the lens of a social public health', *American Journal of Public Health*, 102: 789–99.

Knight, R., Small, W., Carson, A., and Shoveller, J. (2016) 'Complex and conflicting social norms: Implications for implementation of future HIV pre-exposure prophylaxis (PrEP) interventions in Vancouver, Canada', *PLoS One*, 11: e0146513.

Kojima, N., Davey, D.J., and Klausner, J.D. (2016) 'Pre-exposure prophylaxis for HIV infection and new sexually transmitted infections among men who have sex with men', *AIDS*, 30: 2251–2.

Kurth, A.E., Celum, C., Baeten, J.M., Vermund, S.H., and Wasserheit, J.N. (2011) 'Combination HIV prevention: Significance, challenges, and opportunities', *Current HIV/AIDS Reports*, 8: 62–72.

Lasry, A., Sansom, S.L., Wolitski, R.J., Green, T.A., Borkowf, C.B., Patel, P., et al. (2014) 'HIV sexual transmission risk among serodiscordant couples: Assessing the effects of combining prevention strategies', *AIDS*, 28: 1521–9.

Leese, J., Geldman, J., Zhu, S., Macdonald, G.G., Pourrahmat, M.M., Townsend, A.F., et al. (2022) 'Perspectives of persons with arthritis on the use of wearable technology to self monitor physical activity: A qualitative evidence synthesis', *Arthritis Care & Research*, 74: 1520–32.

Makhema, J., Wirth, K.E., Pretorius Holme, M., Gaolathe, T., Mmalane, M., Kadima, E., et al. (2019) 'Universal testing, expanded treatment, and incidence of HIV infection in Botswana', *New England Journal of Medicine*, 381: 230–42.

Marková, I. (1987) 'On the interaction of opposites in psychological processes', *Journal for the Theory of Social Behaviour*, 17(3): 279–99. https://doi.org/10.1111/j.1468-5914.1987.tb00100.x

Marková, I. (2003) *Dialogicality and Social Representations – The Dynamics of Mind*, Cambridge: Cambridge University Press.

Marrazzo, J.M., Ramjee, G., Richardson, B.A., Gomez, K., Mgodi, N., Nair, G., et al. (2015) 'Tenofovir-based preexposure prophylaxis for HIV infection among African women', *New England Journal of Medicine*, 372: 509–18.

Matambanadzo, P., Busza, J., Mafaune, H., Chinyanganya, L., Machingura, F., Ncube, G., et al. (2021) ' "It went through the roof": An observation study exploring the rise in PrEP uptake among Zimbabwean female sex workers in response to adaptations during Covid-19', *Journal of the International AIDS Society*, 24: e25813.

Matswetu, V.S. and Bhana, D. (2018) 'Humhandara and hujaya: Virginity, culture, and gender inequalities among adolescents in Zimbabwe', *Sage Open*, 8: 2158244018779107.

Ministry of Health and Child Care (2018) *Implementation Plan for HIV Pre-Exposure Prophylaxis in Zimbabwe 2018–2020*, Harare, Zimbabwe: Ministry of Health and Child Care.

Ministry of Health and Child Care (2021) *Zimbabwe Population-Based HIV Impact Assessment 2020 (ZIMPHIA 2020): Final Report*, Harare: Ministry of Health and Child Care, Available from: https://phia.icap.columbia.edu/wp-content/uploads/2023/09/010923_ZIMPHIA2020-interactive-versionFinal.pdf [Accessed 22 August 2024].

Ministry of Health and Child Care & National AIDS Council (2020) *Zimbabwe National HIV and AIDS Strategic Plan 2021–2025*, Harare: Ministry of Health and Child Care.

Minkler, M. and Wallerstein, N. (2003) *Community-Based Participatory Research for Health*, San Francisco: John Wiley.

Moorhouse, L., Schaefer, R., Thomas, R., Nyamukapa, C., Skovdal, M., Hallett, T., et al. (2019) 'Application of the HIV prevention cascade to identify, develop, and evaluate interventions to improve use of prevention methods: Examples from a study in east Zimbabwe', *Journal of the International AIDS Society* (submitted).

REFERENCES

Morgan, E., Dyar, C., Newcomb, M.E., D'Aquila, R.T., and Mustanski, B. (2020) 'PrEP use and sexually transmitted infections are not associated longitudinally in a cohort study of young men who have sex with men and transgender women in Chicago', *AIDS and Behavior*, 24: 1334–41.

Moscovici, S. (1973) 'Foreword', in C. Herzlich (ed), *Health and Illness: A Social Psychological Analysis*, London: Academic Press [for] the European Association of Experimental Social Psychology, pp ix–xiv.

Moscovici, S. and Marková, I. (2000) 'Ideas and their development, a dialogue between Serge Moscovici and Ivana Marková', in G. Duveen (ed), *Social Representations, Explorations in Social Psychology*, Cambridge: Polity Press, pp 224–86.

Mowlabocus, S. (2020) '"What a skewed sense of values": Discussing PrEP in the British press', *Sexualities*, 23: 1343–61.

Murchu, E.O., Marshall, L., Teljeur, C., Harrington, P., Hayes, C., Moran, P., et al. (2022) 'Oral pre-exposure prophylaxis (PrEP) to prevent HIV: A systematic review and meta-analysis of clinical effectiveness, safety, adherence and risk compensation in all populations', *BMJ Open*, 12: e048478.

Nelson, G. and Evans, S.D. (2014) 'Critical community psychology and qualitative research: A conversation', *Qualitative Inquiry*, 20: 158–66.

NHS England (2016) 'August update on the commissioning and provision of pre-exposure prophylaxis (PREP) for HIV prevention', Available from: https://www.england.nhs.uk/2016/08/august-update-on-the-commissioning-and-provision-of-pre-exposure-prophylaxis-prep-for-hiv-prevention/ [Accessed 2 August 2016].

Nicolini, D. (2009) 'Zooming in and out: Studying practices by switching theoretical lenses and trailing connections', *Organization Studies*, 30: 1391–418.

Nielsen, B. (2023) 'Antallet af nye hivtilfælde er faldet massivt efter "hiv-p-pille": "Det er en kæmpe success"', Danmarks Radio, Available from: https://www.dr.dk/nyheder/indland/antallet-af-nye-hivtilfaelde-er-faldet-massivt-efter-hiv-p-pille-det-er-en-kaempe [Accessed 6 August 2024].

Oswald, F. (2024) 'Anti-fatness in the Ozempic era: State of the landscape and considerations for future research', Fat Studies, 13(4): 1–7.

Pickles, M., Gregson, S., Moorhouse, L., Dadirai, T., Dzamatira, F., Mandizvidza, P., et al. (2023) 'Strengthening the HIV prevention cascade to maximise epidemiological impact in eastern Zimbabwe: A modelling study', *The Lancet Global Health*, 11: e1105–e1113.

Powell, M. (2019) *Understanding the Mixed Economy of Welfare*, Bristol: Policy Press.

Primdahl, N., Borchmann, O., Hanghøj, C., Vincentz Jensen, M., and Skovdal, M. (2022) *PrEPping sundhedstiltag rettet mod HIV-forbyggelse i Danmark – Et vindue ind i hvordan målgruppen og sundhedspersonale oplever og erfarer PrEP*, Copenhagen: University of Copenhagen, Available from: https://publichealth.ku.dk/about-the-department/hsr/research/prepping-health-services-in-denmark/news/stakeholder-report-published/ [Accessed 14 November 2024].

Primdahl, N. and Skovdal, M. (2023) 'The workings of pre-exposure prophylaxis (PrEP) citizenship amongst queer men in Denmark', *Kvinder, Køn & Forskning*, 35: 102–17.

Primdahl, N.L., Nached, A., and Skovdal, M. (2021) 'Socio-ethical considerations in peer research with newly arrived migrant and refugee young people in Denmark: Reflections from a peer researcher', *Peer Research in Health and Social Development*, Abingdon: Routledge, pp 163–75.

Punchihewa, T.M., Wiles, J., and Saxton, P.J.W. (2024) 'More than prevention: Early adoption of HIV pre-exposure prophylaxis (PrEP) by gay and bisexual men in New Zealand', *Culture, Health & Sexuality*, 26: 222–35.

Rao, A., Moorhouse, L., Maswera, R., Dadirai, T., Mandizvidza, P., Nyamukapa, C., et al. (2022) 'Status of the HIV epidemic in Manicaland, east Zimbabwe prior to the outbreak of the COVID-19 pandemic', *PLoS One*, 17: e0273776.

Rogers, B.G., Coats, C.S., Adams, E., Murphy, M., Stewart, C., Arnold, T., et al. (2020) 'Development of telemedicine infrastructure at an LGBTQ+ clinic to support HIV prevention and care in response to COVID-19, Providence, RI', *AIDS and Behavior*, 24: 2743–7.

Rolle, C.P., Rosenberg, E.S., Siegler, A.J., Sanchez, T.H., Luisi, N., Weiss, K., et al. (2017) 'Challenges in translating PrEP interest into uptake in an observational study of young black MSM', *Journal of Acquired Immune Deficiency Syndromes*, 76: 250–8.

Rubem da Silva-Brandao, R. and Ianni, A.M.Z. (2024) 'Exploring the HIV pre-exposure prophylaxis (PrEP) risk rituals: Individualisation, uncertainty and social iatrogenesis', *Health, Risk & Society*, 26: 19–36.

Saul, J., Bachman, G., Allen, S., Toiv, N.F., and Cooney, C. (2018) 'The DREAMS core package of interventions: A comprehensive approach to preventing HIV among adolescent girls and young women', *PLoS One*, 13: e0208167.

Saul, J., Cooney, C., Hosseini, P.R., Beamon, T., Toiv, N., Bhatt, S., et al. (2022) 'Modeling DREAMS impact: Trends in new HIV diagnoses among women attending antenatal care clinics in DREAMS countries', *AIDS*, 36: S51–9.

Schaefer, R., Gregson, S., Eaton, J.W., Mugurungi, O., Rhead, R., Takaruza, A., et al. (2017) 'Age-disparate relationships and HIV incidence in adolescent girls and young women: Evidence from a general-population cohort in Zimbabwe', *AIDS*, 31(10): 1461–70.

Schensul, S., Schensul, J.J., and LeCompte, M.D. (1999) *Essential Ethnographic Methods: Observations, Interviews & Questionnaires (The Ethnographer's Toolkit)*, Walnut Creek: AltaMira Press.

Skovdal, M. (2019) 'Facilitating engagement with PrEP and other HIV prevention technologies through practice-based combination prevention', *Journal of the International AIDS Society*, 22: e25294.

Skovdal, M., Campbell, C., Nyamukapa, C., and Gregson, S. (2011) 'When masculinity interferes with women's treatment of HIV infection: A qualitative study about adherence to antiretroviral therapy in Zimbabwe', *Journal of the International AIDS Society*, 14: 29.

Skovdal, M., Magoge-Mandizvidza, P., Maswera, R., Moyo, M., Nyamukapa, C., Thomas, R., et al. (2021) 'Stigma and confidentiality indiscretions: Intersecting obstacles to the delivery of pre-exposure prophylaxis to adolescent girls and young women in East Zimbabwe', in S. Bernays, A. Bourne, S. Kippax, P. Aggleton, and R. Parker (eds), *Remaking HIV Prevention in the 21st Century: The Promise of TasP, U=U and PrEP*, Cham: Springer International Publishing, pp 237–48.

Skovdal, M., Clausen, C., Magoge-Mandizvidza, P., Dzamatira, F., Maswera, R., Nyamwanza, R., et al. (2022a) 'How gender norms and 'good girl' notions prevent adolescent girls and young women from engaging with PrEP: Qualitative insights from Zimbabwe', *BMC Women's Health*, 22: 344.

Skovdal, M., Magoge-Mandizvidza, P., Dzamatira, F., Maswera, R., Nyamukapa, C., Thomas, R., et al. (2022b) 'Improving access to pre-exposure prophylaxis for adolescent girls and young women: Recommendations from healthcare providers in eastern Zimbabwe', *BMC Infectious Diseases*, 22: 399.

Skovdal, M., Khayinza Sørensen, O.N., Muchemwa, D., Nyamwanza, R.P., Maswera, R., Svendsen, M.N., et al. (2023) ' "It will not be easy to accept": Parents conflicting attitudes towards pre-exposure prophylaxis for HIV prevention amongst adolescent girls and young women', *Research in Social and Administrative Pharmacy*, 19: 266–71.

Smith, D., Herbst, J., Zhang, X., and Rose, C. (2015) 'Condom effectiveness for HIV prevention by consistency of use among men who have sex with men in the United States', *Journal of Acquired Immune Deficiency Syndromes*, 68: 337–44.

Smith, D.K., Sullivan, P.S., Cadwell, B., Waller, L.A., Siddiqi, A., Mera-Giler, R., et al. (2020) 'Evidence of an association of increases in pre-exposure prophylaxis coverage with decreases in human immunodeficiency virus diagnosis rates in the United States, 2012–2016', *Clinical Infectious Diseases*, 71: 3144–51.

REFERENCES

Spieldenner, A. (2016) 'PrEP whores and HIV prevention: The queer communication of HIV pre-exposure prophylaxis (PrEP)', *Journal of Homosexuality*, 63: 1685–97.

Statens Serum Institut (2023) *HIV 2022*.

Stover, J., Bollinger, L., Izazola, J.A., Loures, L., DeLay, P., Ghys, P.D., et al. (2016) 'What is required to end the AIDS epidemic as a public health threat by 2030? The cost and impact of the fast-track approach', *PLoS One*, 11: e0154893.

Sullivan, A.K., Saunders, J., Desai, M., Cartier, A., Mitchell, H.D., Jaffer, S., et al. (2023) 'HIV pre-exposure prophylaxis and its implementation in the PrEP Impact Trial in England: A pragmatic health technology assessment', *The Lancet HIV*, 10: e790–e806.

Taggart, T., Liang, Y., Pina, P., and Albritton, T. (2020) 'Awareness of and willingness to use PrEP among Black and Latinx adolescents residing in higher prevalence areas in the United States', *PLoS One*, 15: e0234821.

Thomas, R., Skovdal, M., Galizzi, M., Schaefer, R., Moorhouse, L., Nyamukapa, C., et al. (2020a) 'Improving risk perception and uptake of pre-exposure prophylaxis (PrEP) through interactive feedback-based counselling with and without community engagement in young women in Manicaland, East Zimbabwe: Study protocol for a pilot randomised trial', *Trials* (https://pubmed.ncbi.nlm.nih.gov/31973744/) [Accessed 14 November 2024].

Thomas, R., Skovdal, M., Galizzi, M.M., Schaefer, R., Moorhouse, L., Nyamukapa, C., et al. (2020b) Improving risk perception and uptake of voluntary medical male circumcision with peer-education sessions and incentives, in Manicaland, East Zimbabwe: Study protocol for a pilot randomised trial, *Trials*, 21: 1–9.

Toska, E., Cluver, L.D., Boyes, M.E., Isaacsohn, M., Hodes, R., and Sherr, L. (2017) 'School, supervision and adolescent-sensitive clinic care: Combination social protection and reduced unprotected sex among HIV-positive adolescents in South Africa', *AIDS and Behavior*, 21: 2746–59.

Traeger, M.W., Guy, R., Asselin, J., Patel, P., Carter, A., Wright, E.J., et al. (2022) 'Real-world trends in incidence of bacterial sexually transmissible infections among gay and bisexual men using HIV pre-exposure prophylaxis (PrEP) in Australia following nationwide PrEP implementation: an analysis of sentinel surveillance data', *The Lancet Infectious Diseases*, 22: 1231–41.

TV2 (2016) 'Etisk Råd-medlem: Kondom bør komme før dyr hiv-behandling', 13 May 2016, Available from: https://nyheder.tv2.dk/samfund/2016-05-13-etisk-raad-medlem-kondom-boer-komme-foer-dyr-hiv-behandling [Accessed 28 November 2024].

UNAIDS (2014) *Fast-Track – Ending the AIDS Epidemic by 2030*, Geneva: Joint United Nations Programme on HIV/AIDS.

UNAIDS (2019) *Women and HIV: A Spotlight on Adolescent Girls and Young Women*, Geneva: UNAIDS.

UNAIDS (2022a) *HIV Prevention 2025 Road Map – Getting on Track to End AIDS as a Public Health Threat by 2030*, Geneva: Joint United Nations Programme on HIV/AIDS.

UNAIDS (2022b) *In Danger: UNAIDS Global AIDS Update 2022*, Geneva: Joint United Nations Programme on HIV.

UNAIDS (2023) *The Path That Ends AIDS: 2023 UNAIDS Global AIDS Update*, Geneva: Joint United Nations Programme on HIV/AIDS.

Van Damme, L., Corneli, A., Ahmed, K., Agot, K., Lombaard, J., Kapiga, S., et al. (2012) 'Preexposure prophylaxis for HIV infection among African women', *New England Journal of Medicine*, 367: 411–22.

von Schreeb, S., Pedersen, S.K., Christensen, H., Jørgsensen, K.M., Harritshøj, L.H., Hertz, F.B., et al. (2024) 'Questioning risk compensation: Pre-exposure prophylaxis (PrEP) and sexually transmitted infections among men who have sex with men, capital region of Denmark, 2019 to 2022', *Eurosurveillance*, 29: 2300451.

Wang, C. and Burris, M. (1997) 'Photovoice: Concept, methodology, and use for participatory needs assessment', *Health Education & Behaviour*, 24: 369–87.

REFERENCES

Ward, H., Garnett, G.P., Mayer, K.H., and Dallabetta, G.A. (2019) 'Maximizing the impact of HIV prevention technologies in sub-Saharan Africa', *Journal of the International AIDS Society*, 22: e25319.

Wellings, K., Collumbien, M., Slaymaker, E., Singh, S., Hodges, Z., Patel, D., et al. (2006) 'Sexual behaviour in context: a global perspective', *The Lancet*, 368: 1706–28.

WHO (2022) *Differentiated and Simplified Pre-Exposure Prophylaxis for HIV Prevention: Update to WHO Implementation Guidance*, Geneva: World Health Organisation, Available from: https://www.who.int/publications/i/item/9789240053694 [Accessed 9 November 2023].

Wood, S., Dowshen, N., Bauermeister, J.A., Lalley-Chareczko, L., Franklin, J., Petsis, D., et al. (2020) 'Social support networks among young men and transgender women of color receiving HIV pre-exposure prophylaxis', *Journal of Adolescent Health*, 66: 268–74.

Yin, K., Jung, J., Coiera, E., Laranjo, L., Blandford, A., Khoja, A., et al. (2020) 'Patient work and their contexts: Scoping review', *Journal of Medical Internet Research*, 22: e16656.

Yin, R.K. (2003) *Case Study Research: Design and Methods*, Thousand Oaks: Sage Publications.

Young, I., Flowers, P., and McDaid, L. (2016) 'Can a pill prevent HIV? Negotiating the biomedicalisation of HIV prevention', *Sociology of Health & Illness*, 38: 411–25.

Zapata, J.P., Petroll, A., de St. Aubin, E., and Quinn, K. (2022) 'Perspectives on social support and stigma in PrEP-related care among gay and bisexual men: A qualitative investigation', *Journal of Homosexuality*, 69: 254–76.

Zimbabwe National Statistics Agency (2022) *2022 Population and Housing Census. Preliminary Report on Population Figures*, Available from: https://www.zimstat.co.zw/wp-content/uploads/2022/07/Census2022_Preliminary_Report.pdf [Accessed 22 August 2024].

Index

90-90-90/95-95-95 targets 6–7, 32

A

abandonment, risk of 46, 117, 124
addiction 129, 139, 140
adherence difficulties 130–5
adherence levels 8, 134
advocacy 52
agency, of PrEP pill 14
'AIDS-competent community' 151
AIDS-Fondet 31
anonymisation 40
antiretroviral treatment 6, 45, 66, 109–10, 112
apps
  dating apps 79, 80, 82–5, 86, 92, 95
  pill-taking apps 131
Attride-Stirling, J. 41
Auerbach, J.D. 12, 148
Australia 8, 150
Auvert, B. 6

B

Bagge-Petersen, C.M. 14
balancing side-effects with benefits 107–11
battle of ideas 19–21, 145, 147
Bernays, S. 10
Bhana, D. 28
Bill and Melinda Gates Foundation 8–9

Billig, M. 19, 20
biomedical innovation 9
biomedical prevention 3–5
Birk, H. 30
Brisson, J. 14
Bui, H.N. 28

C

Cambiano, V. 16
Campbell, C. 148, 151
caps on funding 69
Carpentier, F.R.D. 95
casual sex 78, 80, 82, 95, 129
centralised PrEP services 32, 42, 54–7, 146
Checkpoint 30
check-ups 85, 102
chemsex 114, 118–21, 125
Chibango, V. 28
choice of methods 9
circumcision 6
Cluver, L.D. 11
co-construction of new norms 149
cognitive polyphasia 19–20, 152
Cohen, M.S. 6
Cold Spring Harbour Laboratory 8–9
collaborative data analysis 41
collectivist cultures 68, 76
combination HIV prevention 11, 16
community health psychology research 25

INDEX

community identity 71, 150
community-based interventions 10–12
community-level awareness 29
comparative case study method 31–5
complexity theory 11
condom use
  access to condoms in Zimbabwe 80, 81
  availability to young women 124
  as cheaper alternative to PrEP 51
  difficulties in consistent use of 78, 80
  negotiating condom use 80–2, 83–4, 115
  'othering' 93
  responsibility for 16
  statistics 6
condomless sex
  chemsex 119
  concerns about PrEP leading to more 16, 44
  detailing *past* history of 88, 89
  eligibility criteria 33, 88, 89
  'othering' of non-PrEP users 93
  PrEP enables 82, 85, 91, 95, 140
  PrEP status signals an interest in 83, 87
  sexually transmitted infections in general 44, 82, 84, 85, 86, 146
confidentiality 29, 134
contraceptives 9
controversies around PrEP 14–17, 19, 30, 42, 51–2, 58, 88, 130, 133, 154
Corbin, J. 13
cost of PrEP 15, 26, 30, 32, 48–59, 146, 153
cost-benefit analysis 107–11, 120, 143
cost-effectiveness 16, 54–8, 69–70, 103
covert use of PrEP 67–8, 116–17, 133–5, 140–1
cover-up for treatment, PrEP seen as 66
COVID-19 10
critical dialogue 148–9

critical social research 24–5
cultural eligibility 61, 64, 69, 76

D

daily pill-taking, difficulties in 130–5
data analysis 40–1
data collection 36
dating apps 79, 80, 82–5, 86, 92, 95
Dean, T. 14
deaths from HIV statistics 5
decentralised PrEP provision 32, 153
Demetriou, D.Z. 29
Denmark
  case study 29–31
  free PrEP 33, 48
  HIV close to eliminated 32
  incidence of sexually-transmitted infections 17
  prevalence of HIV 29, 31
  prevalence of PrEP 30–1
  previous studies 13
  summary of PrEP services 33–4
dependency on male partners 53, 58, 107, 128
dependency on PrEP 128–9, 140
deservedness 48, 52
Determined, Resilient, Empowered, AIDS- free, Mentored, and Safe (DREAMS) 11–12
differentiated health service provision 10, 57
disclosing PrEP status 83, 87, 95, 132–3, 134, 141
disclosures required to access PrEP 14, 89, 95, 103, 127, 132
discontinuing PrEP 135–9, 140
discretion in taking PrEP 67–8
  see also hiding use of PrEP
'do no harm' principle 71
documentaries 15
drugs (chemsex) 114, 118–21
dual prevention pills (PrEP and contraceptives) 9
Durand-Zaleski, I. 16

E

effectiveness of PrEP 7, 114
eligibility criteria
   Denmark 32, 33, 51
   healthy kidneys 122
   PrEP as public health good 104
   queer communities redefining 70–1, 103
   screening processes 51, 88, 89, 97, 103, 122, 146
   shift from past to future risk 44, 72, 146, 149
   unmarried women's eligibility for PrEP 61–2
   vulnerability as eligibility criteria 70, 71, 74
   Zimbabwe 26, 33
eligible, yet ineligible paradox 43, 60–77, 143
Ellis, C. 25
embarrassment 70
   see also shame
epidemic control 5–7
ethics approvals 27, 31
Evans, S.D. 25
everyday living, PrEP working in 12–14
'everyday PrEP negotiations' 2, 19–21, 42–7, 70–5, 125, 129–30, 143, 146–7, 152
existential transformation 127–8, 136, 139–40
extramarital sex 61–3, 145
   see also unfaithfulness

F

Farr, R. 19
Fast-Track approach 6–7
fear of accessing clinics 68
fees for accessing PrEP 53–4
feminist research 24–5
fertility effects 123
Fidan, A. 28
Flyvbjerg, B. 4
focus group discussions 35–6
Food and Drug Administration 15
Food and Drug Administration (US) 15
free, yet costly paradox 42, 48–59, 143
free PrEP 15, 26, 30, 32, 42, 48, 103, 143, 145
freedom, PrEP provides 23, 47, 99, 118–19, 126–41
   see also liberating, yet constraining paradox
frequency of PrEP service 34
Frescura, L. 6

G

Gammeltoft, T.M. 14
García-Iglesias, J. 14
gender norms
   hegemonic masculinity 28–9
   resulting in stigma of PrEP 76
   risks of violence/abandonment 117, 124
   social risks 115–18, 149
   Zimbabwe culture 28–9, 46, 53, 124, 145
   see also 'good girl' norms; patriarchy
generic drugs 15
geographical accessibility 53, 54–5
Giovenco, D. 149
global targets to address HIV 5–7, 32
'good girl' norms 43, 61–5, 69, 76, 115, 117, 124, 144–5
Gourlay, A. 12
Gregson, S. 124, 149
Grindr 82–3, 86, 92, 95

H

Haaland, I. 13
Haggerty, T. 154
Haire, B. 150
Harawa, N.T. 17
harmful sexual activity 46, 103, 114, 115, 118–21
Hawkes, N. 15
Hayes, R.J. 7
health economists 30, 51, 103
health maintenance 99, 102–7
health service capacity 10
health sociology 13

INDEX

healthy, yet a patient paradox 45, 97–113, 143
Hedrick, A.M. 95
hegemonic masculinity 28–9
heteronormativity 147
heterosexual women and the effectiveness of PrEP 8
hiding use of PrEP 67–8, 116–17, 133–5, 140–1
HIV background 5–7
HIV infection statistics 5, 7
hookups 78, 80, 95
Hoppe, T.A. 12, 148
hospital-based services 30, 55, 97–8, 100–2, 105, 132, 151
hospital/consultation fees 53–4

I

Ianni, A.M.Z. 125
illness-related work 13
impact maximisation 8–12
Impact Trial (UK) 15
implants 9
indiscretion 67–8
individual versus society's responsibility for risk 15, 17, 30
infections with HIV, statistics 5, 7
infectious disease departments 30, 55, 97–8, 100–2
infidelity 45, 61, 76, 81, 106, 109, 115, 145
informal networks 90
injectable PrEP 9
internalised homophobia 117, 128, 145
International AIDS Conference (19th) in Washington 5–6
interview methods 35–6, 38–40
intimate partner violence 28, 116, 117
'invincibility' 138–9
Iwuji, C.C. 7

J

Joffe, H. 18
Joint United Nations Programme on HIV/AIDS 26
Jovchelovitch, S. 19

K

Kambarami, M. 28
Katz, A.W.K. 149
kidney function 1, 33, 34, 122
Kippax, S. 12, 153
Knight, R. 2
Kojima, N. 16
Kurth, A.E. 11

L

Lasry, A. 16
legitimation of queer sex 128
lenient service providers 74
liberating, yet constraining paradox 47, 126–41, 143, 150
'lifestyle drugs' 16
lived experience 36, 39–40
liver function 123
locations for PrEP service 10–11, 34, 67–8, 153
 see also hospital-based services; infectious disease departments
longer-acting PrEP 9
long-term effects 46, 114, 121–3, 138
'luxury' problems 131, 132
lying 43, 61, 69–75, 76–7, 134, 148–9

M

Makhema, J. 7
Manicaland, Zimbabwe 27–8
marketing and health campaigns 153
Marková, I. 19, 20, 152
Matambanadzo, P. 11, 26
Matswetu, V.S. 28
meaning-making 150–1
men of colour 8
men who have sex with men
 effectiveness of PrEP 7
 heterogeneity 8
 prevalence of STIs 16
mental work 144, 151, 154
meta-analyses 7
Moorhouse, L. 23

moral responsibilities 14–17, 30, 44, 65, 144–8
Morgan, E. 16
mortality rates 5
Moscovici, S. 18, 19
Mowlabocus, S. 15, 16
multiple sexual partners 89
  see also promiscuity
Murchu, E.O. 7, 8, 16, 78
'My PrEP Experience' 95

N

National AIDS Trust 15
national health services 15, 17, 30, 48, 50, 56, 71
Nelson, G. 25
Nguyen, V.-K. 14
NHS England 15–16
Nicolini, D. 35
number/statistic, feeling reduced to 104–5
Nyamwanza, Rangarirayi Primrose 40

O

observational data 36
online procurement of PrEP 123
open relationships 136–9
opening hours 55, 57, 153
opportunity costs of accessing PrEP 54–7, 132
Oswald, F. 154
'othering' 44, 67, 86, 92–4, 143, 150
out-of-pocket expenses 48–9, 53–4

P

parents' attitudes
  disapproval of PrEP use 43, 60, 62–5, 68, 115–16, 140
  premarital/extramarital sex 28–9, 62–3
  promising not to contract HIV 71
  risk of abandonment by parents 46
  risk of parents finding out supersedes benefits of PrEP 68
  social control 115–16, 140, 145
  supportive 124, 149

participant characteristics 36, 37
participant recruitment 36
participatory research methodologies 25, 27, 31
partners
  attitudes to PrEP use 60, 64, 68, 115–16, 124, 145
  disclosing PrEP to 133
  discussing PrEP use with 75, 116–17, 138, 141
  hiding use of PrEP from 67–8, 116–17, 133–5, 140–1
  intimate partner violence 28, 116, 117
  protection from risky behaviour of 94, 106
  social risks 115–18
  unfaithfulness 45, 61, 76, 81, 106, 109, 115, 145
  Zimbabwean women's dependency on male partners 53, 58, 107, 128
patient, being a 97–113, 143
patient work 13–14, 111, 130, 135, 144, 154–5
patriarchy 17, 28–9, 46, 115, 124, 145, 146–7
peer research 40
People vs The NHS: Who Gets the Drugs? 15
pharmacies 56, 103
Photovoice 27, 31, 35–6, 38, 39
Pickles, M. 16
'Picturing PrEP' exhibition 38–9
pillboxes 131–2
pill-taking norms 98–9, 102, 109–10, 112, 130–5
pill-taking work 130–5, 140, 144
policy frameworks 69–75
population-level reductions in new HIV infections 7
post-humanism 14
Potgieter, C. 28
poverty 27, 53, 146
Powell, M. 35
power
  negotiating condom use 80–2, 115
  research process 24–6
  'PrEP-competent social networks' 151, 153

INDEX

prevalence of HIV
 Danish case study 29, 31
 Zimbabwe case study 27
prevention targets 6–7
preventive medicine as a field 3–5, 153–5
price of drugs 15
Primdahl, N.L. 13, 14, 40, 41
privilege, PrEP as 49–53, 55
productive role of paradoxes 151–3
promiscuity 15, 16, 30, 44, 63, 78, 79–80, 88, 145, 146
public health good, PrEP as 52, 58, 71, 103, 104, 105, 107, 111
Punchihewa, T.M. 139

Q

qualitative studies 27
queer rights 52

R

Rao, A. 27
religion 63
remembering to take pills 131
research process 24–6, 35–47
research stance 24–6
responsible, yet irresponsible paradox 44, 78–96, 143, 150
risk
 of abandonment 46, 117, 124
 focus on past risk over future 146
 individual versus society's responsibility for risk 15, 17, 30
 long-term effects 121–3
 PrEP enables risky behaviours 120
 protection from partner's risky behaviour 94, 106
 responsibility for 15, 17, 30, 44, 70
 risky behaviour as eligibility criteria 71–2, 146
 shift from past to future risk 44, 72, 146, 149
 social risks 46, 68, 115–18, 124, 133, 147

risks of PrEP itself 46, 114
 see also side-effects
Rolle, C.P. 8
Rubem da Silva-Brandao, R. 125

S

safe, yet unsafe paradox 46, 114–25
safety/comfort, PrEP as 71, 143
Saksom community 27
sampling 36
Saul, J. 11
Schaefer, R. 28
Schensul, S. 35
screening processes 51, 88, 89, 97, 103, 122, 146
secret use of PrEP 67–8, 116–17, 133–5, 140–1
self-care, PrEP as 105–7
self-funded PrEP 16
sense-making 20, 58, 113, 143, 148–9
serodiscordant couples 7
service packages for PrEP 34
sex workers 11, 26, 65–6, 145
sexual activity
 casual sex 78, 80, 82, 95, 129
 chemsex 114, 118–21, 125
 eligibility criteria 71–4
 fears that PrEP may augment harmful 118–21
 harmful sexual activity 46, 103, 114, 115, 118–21
 'othering' 92
 partners' 106
 premarital/extramarital sex 28–9, 62–3
 PrEP enables potentially risky behaviours 82, 85, 91, 95, 140
 responsible, yet irresponsible 78–96
 shame over 88
 see also condomless sex; promiscuity; unprotected sex
sexual capital 87, 149–50
sexual freedom 47, 127–30, 136–9, 150
sexual health 78–96

Printed and bound by CPI Group (UK) Ltd, Croydon, CR0 4YY
17/11/2025

14774038-0001